FEAST & FAMINE

HEALING ADDICTION WITH GRACE

ROBIN H. CLARE

FEAST & FAMINE

Quantity sales special discounts are available on quantity purchases by corporations, associations, and others. For details, contact the publisher at the address above.

Orders by U.S. trade bookstores and wholesalers. Email info@ BeyondPublishing.net

The Beyond Publishing Speakers Bureau can bring authors to your live event. For more information or to book an event contact the Beyond Publishing Speakers Bureau speak@BeyondPublishing.net

The Author can be reached directly at info@clare-ity.com

Manufactured and printed in the United States of America distributed globally by BeyondPublishing.net

BEYOND
PUBLISHING

New York | Los Angeles | London | Sydney

ISBN Hardcover: 978-1-949873-74-0

ISBN Softcover: 978-1-949873-79-5

This book is dedicated to:

Kathleen Humpage

You have graced my life with your profound wisdom.

One beautiful summer evening I was walking my dog,
Hailey, in our neighborhood and we were the only ones
on the street. The air was utterly still, and I knew that the
Divine was close by.

I looked up at the heavens and knew that the next words
out of my mouth would be my most sacred admission.
Hesitantly, I said " I am afraid that if I surrender my life to
Divine service, you will not provide for me."

God replied, "My dear, Robin, did you know that "dog" is
"God" spelled backwards?"
I laughed and said, " I think I read that somewhere."

God spoke again, "Think of yourself as your dog and think of
us as you. Is there anything that you would not do for your
precious dog because of your shared unconditional love?"

I replied, " I would do anything for Hailey,"
God replied, "And we would do anything for you."

CONTENTS

When Robin shared with me that she was guided to write a book with Sophia, the Universal Mother on our global addiction problem, I was not surprised. Robin has displayed the courage and openness to take on writing assignments that others would shy away from. "Suffering is the only addiction on our planet," says Sophia to Robin in *Feast & Famine*. Then, we choose a tool to perpetuate the pain – like substances or vices. By connecting to Sophia (recognized as heavenly grace), humanity can heal their individual and collective suffering. Discover how to surrender and allow grace into your life. Brilliant!

James Twyman, *New York Times Best-Selling Author, and Award-Winning Filmmaker*

What a gem! *Feast & Famine* by Robin Clare is not just another book on addictions. This book includes inspiration, practical advice, Robin's account of her 40-year struggle with bulimia, and most amazingly, channeled messages from Sophia, the Divine Universal Mother. Through Robin, Sophia outlines her Divine Healing Path so one can move from addiction, in any form, to recovery. An exciting and easy read on such a serious and relevant topic.

Dolores Arsenault, *Future Author of Trusting the Guru Within*

"Highly recommended! Robin Clare reveals the secret to all addictions in this evocative and inspiring account of how she overcame her lifelong struggle with eating disorders. *Feast & Famine* is a must-read for all who struggle with addictions!

Randy Peyser, *Author of The Power of Miracle Thinking*

Robin Clare's *Feast & Famine* frank and fascinating exploration of addiction and recovery from a personal, practical, and spiritual standpoint is a powerful asset in tackling your own "suffering." This book makes clear that our core wounds—our suffering—is all the same addiction –it's just a matter which tool you use to self-medicate. This book chronicles Robin's struggle with bulimia, and whatever your drug of choice, you'll see yourself in its pages. Guided by the spirit of the Divine Universal Mother, working through Robin, you'll see addiction—and the recovery process--through new eyes and an open heart.

Jackie Lapin, Author of Practical Conscious Creation:
Daily Techniques to Manifest Your Dreams

Bravo! I loved, loved, loved *Feast & Famine* the first and second time I read it! The most profound message I took from the book was that if we are not living in grace, then we are suffering. Let's say that again; If we are not living in grace, then we are suffering. No more hiding from this truth or ourselves. The idea that we either choose grace OR suffering is so simple and divine.

Kristine Burke, Founder, MasterfulU

In her latest book, *Feast & Famine*, Robin Clare writes, "*The Divine is only one breath away, waiting, and wanting to help each one of us live our most happy lives.*" What an amazing and uplifting statement to read at the beginning of a book about addiction! Hopeful is the best word I can use to describe this vulnerable and courageous work, based on her own life's struggle with food addiction. As Robin goes on to explain, many humans are addicted to suffering; then, we choose the vehicle which works best to keep us in that state. Her belief that maybe when we learn the reasoning behind our favorite brand of suffering, we can recover from it, is refreshing and intelligent, wholly hopeful.

Lowri Foyle, Future Author of Playing the Game:
Self-Help for Kids (Of All Ages) with Gaming Issues

Feast & Famine is a chronicle of Robin's profound journey to and through recovery, supported by her Sophia, the Divine Universal Mother. This book is a beautiful mainline shot to the Divine, acknowledging that we are all recovering from something. I applaud Robin for her soulful candor and kind teaching by revealing the gifts of suffering. The healing narrative infuses the reader with love and grace.

Amy LaBossiere, Author of Finding Still Waters:
The Art of Conscious Recovery

Robin has crafted an excellent book that any addict can relate to. I'm a recovering drug addict and alcoholic myself, sober since 1985. I remembered my struggles with emotional pain and suffering in addiction while reading about Robin's story because I can relate. I love this book because she *wholeheartedly* brings us through the pain of addiction to the Light of recovery while partnering with Divine Guidance. I loved the (obviously) cleaver insights inserted by Sophia. Thank you, Robin, for this amazing gift of a book. Your courage and vulnerability of sharing your journey is an inspiration to me. It was a reminder that no one of us needs to suffer. And we're all in this *recovery* . . . together.

Maureen Ross Gemme, MS Ed., Author of Emerge: 7 Steps to Transformation (No Matter What Life Throws At You!)

Robin's book is a blessing of light and grace for all of us who share the very human path of addictive suffering while simultaneously being on our unique spiritual path. Robin's story is augmented by the wisdom and compassion of her special Divine guest~Sophia. *Feast & Famine* offers a gentle yet powerful approach to healing your past, coming to terms with your present, and surrendering resistance to resonating with your clearest, healthiest, and best-empowered self. Read this book to discover the hidden gems within!

Valerie Coleman-Palansky, LCSW, MS Ed, LMT, Energy-Based Teacher and Healer

Not only is *Feast & Famine* engaging, but the content resonated deeply and sparked epiphanies within me. In this pure, yet compelling book, Robin, gently invites each one of us to accept that suffering is a natural human condition and to achieve transformation from this condition, we need to embrace our Divinity. Robin demonstrates personal courage and grace as she shares her extraordinary experiences. By understanding the teachings within this powerful book, you will open your heart to compassion for self and others and healing of self and all of humanity.

Karina Viante-Phelan, Founder of Crystal Stream Healing LLC & Divine By Design

FOREWORD

An Artist's Statement

Robin and I sat in a coffee shop discussing her new book, *Feast & Famine: Healing Addiction with Grace.*

We are old friends, and she knows me not only as an artist but also as a person in recovery from addiction and who coaches others in recovery. She knows that I understand the addiction and recovery process in general and that I have battled food addiction even in recovery from substance addiction.

We discussed several approaches the cover illustration could take, and back in the studio, I tried several. None quite hit the mark. There was something key that was missing, and we could not quite get a handle on it. Then she intuited an idea that we instantly recognized as the solution: we needed to illustrate the brokenness a person feels in addiction and what it takes to feel whole again.

Through several more discussions and sketches, we came to the current design: a representation of kintsugi, the Japanese art of ceramic repair that uses precious metal to "heal" the broken pieces. Kintsugi teaches that the "scars" add beauty to the object and that broken objects are not something to hide but to display with pride.

In recovery from addiction, our wounds each have their own story and beauty, once we learn the grace that lies hidden within them.

Uncovering the traumas that cause addiction and are caused by it, learning from the experiences, and realizing that these experiences are what make each person unique and precious: this is the essence of resilience.

For me, the inner reflection involved in creating this cover was a reminder that even in recovery, I continue to break at times, as we all do. Having a book like this to *gracefully* guide us back to wholeness is a true gift.

Thank you, Robin, for bringing us this gift.

George Herrick, *Life Coach and Artist*

PREFACE

Sophia came face-to-face with me at the end of a healing session while I was in a meditative state. In my meditation, I had just emerged from a cleansing waterfall, and I stood in the still water at its base. A beautiful Being of Light came walking towards me.

She said, "I am Sophia."

I wanted to bow my head in reverence, but I could not take my eyes off her face.

When she first stepped in front of me, her face was one of a young maiden, then she aged before my eyes through every stage of a women's life, including becoming an elder. It seemed that she was every woman merged into one Being of Light. I quickly said to myself, "Stop staring and listen; she must have something important to tell you."

Sophia continued, "I have been speaking to you since you were seventeen years old, preparing you to write this book, and I will be your guide for this book. The name of the book is *Feast & Famine: Healing Addiction with Grace*. This will be your story of addiction and how you have healed your addiction through a deep dedication to your spiritual path."

I had known years ago that I would have to tell my story—to "out" myself to the world—and now the time had arrived. I was not even sure how I felt. Here I was, standing in front of Sophia. How blessed was I? Wait, you are not sure because you don't know who Sophia is? No surprise, because Sophia is the most hidden deity in our religious and spiritual culture.

The aspects of Divinity that Sophia represents are critical to our ability to reach our highest spiritual potential and, therefore, she was removed from most religious texts. Sophia is the Divine Feminism aspects of Creation or, more boldly stated, she is the Mother of Creation. Without her grace, humanity cannot stop suffering, heal from addiction, or reach enlightenment. It is time to surrender our suffering and welcome Sophia into our lives.

Robin H. Clare

ACKNOWLEDGMENTS

I believe that our Soul creates a plan prior to our incarnation that will bring all of the experiences and players into our lives that will enable us to fulfill our Soul's mission. My life's play has been filled with a stellar cast of family, friends, a spiritual/wellness support team, and a professional book team that have each enabled me to find the courage and commitment to write this book.

I could try to name everyone, but that would be an unnecessary task. I am confident that you know who you are. Some of you have been influencing my journey for a lifetime, others for a season, and others just for a reason, bringing me to this exact moment in time writing this note. One could question if I am in your life's play or if you are in my life's play. Either way, you have been an integral part of mine, and I thank you with my entire being.

"Wake up, it's time to start the book," said Sophia in an encouraging way. I jumped out of bed and stepped outside of our family home to witness a glorious new day awakening in nature. My eyes immediately went to the beautiful field of green grass covered with a layer of fog. I shifted my gaze left to watch the summer sunrise over the lake, all the while listening to the sounds of birds chirping and the crows cawing like a beautiful country soundtrack. I stood in the wondrous beauty of nature and gathered up my inspiration. Called inside and now sitting at my writing desk, I stared at my computer, struggling with how I was going to write a book that would be so darn personal and revealing.

I began to rationalize; perhaps if I just say it upfront, the thoughts and words will start to flow, and I can get started on the book. So here it is: I have been an addict my entire adult life. And, at the other end of the spiritual spectrum, I am a spiritual author and teacher. I had compressed myself into the middle, between self- loathing and self-love—quite a complication! In reality, my life felt like a frustrating and shameful contradiction. It would take a request, an ultimatum, and a solution from the Divine for me to move into recovery.

In today's world, addiction is not associated with just drugs, alcohol, and cigarettes. We now recognize addiction in other areas of our lives, including food, gambling, sex, cell phones, watching TV, shopping, social media, and others not listed. Addiction has plagued each one of us, directly or indirectly. With the epidemic of addiction in our world, if you don't have some form of addictive behavior or know someone who struggles with some form of addiction, you are probably in denial.

Based on the many forms of addictive behavior in our world, there is a vast audience for this book; yet, I believe that there is a more specific audience for this book. This is a book for those who believe that, even in the throes of addiction, he or she is loved and protected by a profound source of energy. Does this sound like you? On the surface, you struggle with the same frustration, guilt, and shame as all addicts, but on a very deep level, you believe in your own worthiness, and you also believe that you are of the *Light*. You have learned about the *Light* in your religious or spiritual studies. However, in addiction, you diminish your *Light* on purpose because you are afraid of your own *Light*.

This inspiring quote by Marianne Williamson is from her book, *A Return To Love: Reflections on the Principles of A Course in Miracles* and describes my audience perfectly:

> Our deepest fear is not that we are inadequate. Our deepest fear is that we are powerful beyond measure. It is our light, not our darkness that most frightens us. We ask ourselves, Who am I to be brilliant, gorgeous, talented, fabulous? Actually, who are you *not* to be? You are a child of God. Your playing small does not serve the world. There is nothing enlightened about shrinking so that other people won't feel insecure around you. We are all meant to shine, as children do. We were born to make manifest the glory of God that is within us. It's not just in some of us; it's in everyone. And as we let our own light shine, we unconsciously give other people permission to do the same. As we are liberated from our own fear, our presence automatically liberates others.

If you take away one lesson from this book, I hope you come to the ultimate conclusion that you are not alone. The Divine is only one breath away, waiting, and wanting to help each one of us live our most happy lives. Some people refer to the Divine as God or Goddess, as a higher power, as the angels or spirit guides, as nature, as the Universe—and, in fact, they are all correct! By seeing the Divine as a vast resource for my daily life, I have and will live a magical life.

And yet, I am incredibly embarrassed that I have struggled with addiction and its resulting disappointments, shame and guilt. Somehow, I think I should know better, considering who my spiritual mentors are. I have been blessed to write two books with Yeshua (Jesus) and am now guided by Sophia (the Universal Mother) to write this book. Even with these incredible mentors, I remained deeply engaged in my addiction to binging and purging of food (bulimia). Was I unaware that it was an addiction? I have come to understand that any action that you feel compelled to repeat over and over that causes you great suffering is an addiction.

To move into recovery, I had to learn to value my relationship with myself over my relationships with others. I had to learn how to connect to my own inner divinity and then live the spiritual teachings I have received. Since I previously wrote two books on the topic of inner divinity, one would think that it should not have been too hard. My first book, *Messiah Within*, was a guide to living one's inner divinity, and my second book, *The Divine Keys*, was a guidebook on how to achieve a level of magical oneness with the Divine.

I wrote my first two deeply spiritual books as an addict. In fact, I wrote the first draft of this book as an active addict, and it turned out that the ending was kind of lame. It was something like, *I am still an active addict, and I hope you are not. I am not sure if I believe Sophia's path to healing because I am not following it.* Not very inspiring. I knew I had to re-write and publish this book, but that I could not do so until I was in recovery. Honestly, I had no choice; I had to either stop purging or die. Yes, I was scared straight.

What did it take to stop suffering and start loving myself? To stop suffering, I had to surrender. And it was at this point of surrender that Sophia became even more present in my life. Sophia is the facilitator of grace in our lives, and she will come to help us when we are genuinely in surrender. How do you know you are genuinely in surrender? The answer is simple: when you are in surrender, you will see the gift of why you were suffering in the first place.

Like all addicts, I was in a tremendous amount of pain and fear. I had to dig deep into my life to understand the theme of my pain. I had to give up the disappointments, the regrets, and the challenges of the people closest to me throughout my life. I had to learn to love them all in an unconditional manner, which means acceptance without judgment. But most of all, I had to live my life with an integrated system of mind, body, spirit, and emotion.

Let's define what personal success looks like in this balanced, integrated model of living that demonstrates our most magnificent reflection of the Divine. That entails becoming a healthy, creative, compassionate, successful, resourceful, and generous human being. The journey to your everyday wellness will be bumpy, but the destination will be filled with love, peace, joy, and abundance. Thank you for providing me with a forum to share my struggles and my triumphs. If you are reading this book and you are suffering, and in addiction, I appreciate your challenges more than you can know.

While I was preparing to write this book, Sophia said to me, "You know, Robin, there is only ONE addiction in your world."

Now, very curious, I said, "Please, Sophia, share your view."

She said, "This primary addiction is to a life of suffering. What tool you use to satisfy your need to suffer is up to you. Food, alcohol, drugs, sex, social media, cigarettes— you name it— are just the poison one might pick to suffer."

After considering this profound life-changing information that there is only one primary addiction, I asked Sophia, "Why is one addicted to suffering?

*Sophia replied, "The answer is you do not love yourself. Throughout your life, you have learned how **not** to love yourself. For now, let us say that not loving yourself is the problem, and learning to love yourself is the solution to a life without suffering. Let us begin."*

FEAST & FAMINE

A ritual is a sequence of activities involving gestures, words, and objects, performed in a sequestered place, and performed according to set sequence. (Merriam-Webster)

Oh, God, I am really fat tonight.

And then the panic begins. Lying in bed, I begin my evening ritual of judging my body. I start with a careful review of what I ate during the day: was it healthy, was it good for me? And then my thoughts quickly turn to how much did I eat? Did I overeat? Was I bad? I reach for my lower belly and grab my roll of fat to assess (or should I say "obsess"?) how big it is. Then I move to my upper belly to see if it feels bloated. And finally, I reach for my back to see if I have a roll of back fat.

Tonight, the panic is more profound because I will see my family this weekend. I wanted to lose weight for this special event weekend, but I was not successful. I am upset with myself because, in my addict mind, it is too late, so why not just eat whatever the heck I want tonight. I was in the hysteria of dieting for events versus eating for my overall health. And on this particular night, I had no control over how I would respond.

What should I do now?

Can I put on my rational hat and think about all the nutritional food I ate during my day to calm myself down? Or will I spiral down to notice only the extra snacks I ate obsessively after dinner tonight? "The kitchen is closed," said my mother each night of my childhood, to stop us from making a mess in the kitchen, which I, in turn, interpreted as being deprived of food. In researching food deprivation, I learned that inhibiting food intake had consequences that may not have been anticipated by my loved ones. Restrictive dieting appears to result in eating binges once the food is available and in psychological manifestations such as preoccupation with food and eating. Yes, I was utterly preoccupied with food and eating, and the outcomes that would have occurred if I allowed the food to stay in my body on this evening that I am writing about.

The kitchen is closed.

Tonight, I ate all night even after my "kitchen was closed." Was I feeling lonely? Was I hungry? Was I looking for a way to punish myself? Was I rebelling from a childhood rule? Gosh, I am so tired of judging my body, feeling ashamed about blowing my diet, and hearing the scolding from my mother to get out of the kitchen.

"Pull it together, Robin," says the small voice in my head.

I answer, "How can I go to bed with all this food in my belly? I will get fatter." "Don't do it," says the small voice.

On a good night, I will answer, "You're right; tomorrow is another day to get healthy eating right." But not tonight. I lose the battle in my head, and I head to the bathroom where I drink two glasses of water so that my purging will be easier. When I am done, I flush the required number of times to get rid of the evidence. And then I brush my teeth, remembering a strange conversation I had with my father, who was a dentist. Instead of confronting me with what he might have suspected early on, he merely said quietly, "Girls who purge have a greater risk of destroying their tooth enamel."

A lifetime of mixed emotions

I look at myself in the mirror and see the same look on my face that I have seen since I first began binging and purging at seventeen years old. My face is filled with mixed emotions. As I roll my eyes in humiliation, I guiltily wonder what is likely the impact on my internal organs from the purging. I then feel a rationalized sense of relief that now I might not be more fat in the morning.

When I wake up in the morning, I go through the same ritual of judging my body, reaching, and feeling for the rolls of fat. "After all," I think, "it is morning, and I could be thinner." Then my day begins, and the struggle with my food addiction kicks right in. What am I going to have for breakfast? What's for lunch? What am I making for dinner? How many snacks can I eat? Careful not to get too full today, because then I may need to purge. All-day I will think about when I can eat next and what I will eat. I will work hard to balance my nutritional needs with a desire to take off twenty pounds.

Health concerns

Now, I must add in the fact that my cholesterol has gone up, and my blood sugar is elevated. Maybe these two health concerns will be more powerful than my desire to binge and purge. My elevated cholesterol and blood sugar were a direct result of my binging and purging. I've consumed a lot of suger in my adult life. Sugar converts to carbohydrates in the body, resulting in higher cholesterol and blood sugar levels. Why did I eat so much sugar?

In addition to physical addiction, there was another physiological reason why I did so. I discovered that I do not produce dopamine in my brain. Dopamine is the "feel-good" neurotransmitter in the brain. When we have healthy dopamine levels in the brain, we find our inner happiness. When we do not, we look for outside sources (drugs, alcohol, cigarettes, sex, unhealthy relationships, food, TV, social media) to make us feel good. I will address the biology of addiction in greater detail in an upcoming chapter. For now, it is enough to declare that my feel-good drug of choice was food.

It's really about the suffering, not the substances.

Sophia has shared with me that there is only one primary addiction, and that is to suffering. To perpetuate the suffering, we choose substances that facilitate the addictive behavior. So that means, I am primarily addicted to suffering and secondarily addicted to food. That is a tough one to swallow (pun intended). In researching the struggle of addiction, I would read statements like "suffering and struggle are emotional addictions as strong as addictions to alcohol, nicotine, and drugs." If I am correctly interpreting Sophia's statement above, then perhaps there is first an emotional addiction. Then to fulfill that emotional addiction, we must choose a vehicle to sustain the struggling. Even in my own family, I have witnessed various forms of addiction, and, clearly, I have labeled them by their vehicle, not by their source.

Years ago, I was driving into New York with my brother, Michael, who struggled with drug addiction. I turned to him and said, "I think my addiction is worse than yours."

He laughed at me and said, "How can you compare hardcore drugs to food?"

I said, "My drug of choice (food) is in my house and on every street corner in the world. You have to go out and search for your drugs. And besides, it is acceptable for me to use my drug of choice three times a day plus snacks."

We agreed to disagree on that topic. In hindsight, I see now that my addiction to emotional suffering is no better or worse than my brother's addiction to emotional suffering. We had each just chosen different vehicles to express our suffering.

How do we become addicted to suffering? The next chapter offers insights into how we victimize ourselves and the vehicles we use to seek comfort.

"Sophia, which came first, the victim or the addict?" I asked.

Sophia replied, "We would answer 'both.' When you experience hurt by another, you begin to distrust your innate love of self. The moment you begin to loathe yourself, a process starts to perpetuate the victim model. You become addicted to self-hate or loathing of self.

Being the victim and being the addict is so intertwined that the timing is simultaneous, and the emotional impact is the same. And quite often, the victim becomes the victimizer, the one who is hurting himself or herself.

In bulimia, you are both the victim and the victimizer. Your victim is caught in the overeating process, and the victimizer is the one causing you to purge. Being the victim and the victimizer is true for anyone found in any form of addictive behavior."

CHAPTER TWO

VICTIM OR ADDICT

Self-Love is our true nature.

We came into this world as beautiful light beings, all shiny and new and deeply connected to our Divinity. In other words, we came into this world in a state of self-love. Those closest to us (our most essential caregivers) were struggling with their own limited level of self-love. They influenced us and our opinion of ourselves. At birth, we have an innate knowing that "I am Divine." "I am Love." "I am Perfect." Then, our loving caregivers started to compare us to others.

We become subject to our family and societal values and standards, and then we are given our first drug: sugar. Don't many of us find it cute to watch 1-year-olds on their birthday eat a sugary birthday cake? Did we just start them on their path to addiction with a celebration that included a hefty dose of sugar?

The path to addiction begins with childhood trauma.

According to addiction expert Dr. Gabor Maté, the single factor at the core of all addictions is trauma. He describes trauma as "...emotional loss in childhood, and in the case of severe addicts, significant childhood trauma such as family violence, addiction in the family, sexual and emotional abuse, physical abuse, a parent being mentally ill or in jail. These adverse childhood experiences have been shown to exponentially increase the risk of addiction later in life." Dr. Maté further explains in the article "Why This Doctor Believes Addictions Start In Childhood" about another set of painful experiences: when good things don't happen.

A child has certain fundamental needs for emotional development and for brain development. If you look at the human brain, it develops under the impact of the environment. For example, in the case of addiction, the brain's reward circuitry is impaired... the person's circuits, which have to do with the chemical dopamine, and which give you a sense of reward incentive and motivation, are not well-developed. Those circuits need the support of the environment to help them in their development, and the essential quality of the environment is a mutually responsive relationship with the parent or caregiver. Psychological pain at the heart of all addictions and addictive behaviors. Addicts have one intended purpose: to soothe pain or to escape from pain or stress. Whether we're looking at the psychological side of addiction, which is needing to escape from pain or stress, or the brain physiology side, which is the underdeveloped reward circuits in the brain, we're looking at the impact of childhood.

Joy is an inside job.

A naturopath I worked with astutely checked my brain dopamine level. She decided to check my dopamine level due to the obsessive-compulsive nature of my eating disorders. We discovered that my dopamine level was so low that there was no number to report! When the doctor gave me the news, I jumped up and down— finally, a physical reason for why I was looking for joy outside of myself with food. By taking a natural supplement, I have been able to raise my dopamine level. Yet, I know that I cannot forget how much I resonated with being a victim. So which came first, the victim or the addict?

The role of victim in addiction

Kayla Scoumis, in an article titled "Victimhood & Addiction: How to Identify Victim Mentality," describes the victim role as:

> …a way of thinking that essentially makes you feel and act helpless. This type of thinking is dangerous for everyone, but it is especially dangerous for those in active addiction. The victim role allows those in active addiction to manipulate others. The "victims" communicate the beliefs in their head in a way that convinces their friends or loved ones that life truly is as bad as they say. This allows the "victims" to obtain whatever they need to survive in life. In other words, the "victim" manipulates others into enabling him or her.

The article further explains that addicts have adopted the victim mindset because they have been victims of a myriad of traumas. She explains that many individuals define themselves by the tragedy and the trauma that they have experienced. This identity impacts their ability to move forward. Using substances allows these individuals to block emotional pain and feel more comfortable and normal in the world. Once someone translates the trauma into a belief that all they will ever be is a victim of that situation, this then translates to assuming a victim mentality across all areas of life.

Victim or Persecutor, or both

In today's vernacular, we throw the word "victim" around like it's a natural part of life. A victim is defined as a person harmed, injured, or killed because of a crime, accident, or other event or action. But doesn't that sound like someone else is doing something to you? In reality, though, couldn't we be victimizing ourselves by being our own persecutor? A persecutor is defined as a person who harasses or annoys someone persistently. Could that someone be yourself? As an addict, we become our own persecutor, creating harm and injury to ourselves because of our addictive behavior. We want to blame others for our addiction. My mother this, my father that, society this, a religion that.

The bottom line, it is about you hurting yourself. Unless someone is physically forcing you to eat that candy bar, use that needle, pick up your cell phone in the middle of the night to check messages, you are being the persecutor of your own life and making yourself a victim.

A perfect example

It was Christmas Day, and I completely ate like an idiot at my dear friend's holiday party. Of course, there was the voice playing in my head, "Go ahead, eat that, you can always throw up." I listened to that voice in my head, and I overate so much that I became physically ill later that night. My release of all the food was equally physical, as it was emotional and psychological. I had no choice but to be sick. In fact, I believe I overdosed on food that night. I was dizzy; I had pains all over my body; I was sick as a dog. Just a side note: I had zero alcohol. So, my retching was due to my wretched behavior around food. I victimized myself by overeating, and my compulsion was so bad I even got a candy bar when I stopped for gas. Like an alcoholic saying, "Oh, just one more glass of wine."

After this bulimic episode, the lower half of my body was in so much pain. My hips, thighs, knees, and feet were barely working together. When I woke up the next morning, I stared out the window at a beautifully fallen snow and asked myself, "Why do I feel like crap?" Can you guess the answer? "Because you are eating crap," said my intuitive self. The expression, "We are what we eat" is so incredibly accurate. These aches and pains are just warning signs for what a life of living with an illness or long-term self-destruction can feel like.

Is it possible that we have patterns in our lives that set us up for suffering and ultimately addictive behaviors? In the next chapter, we will look at the pattern of humiliation as a driver for addiction.

"Sophia, where does addiction begin?" I asked.

Sophia replied, "Your beginning is that moment when you first experienced disappointment or heartache from someone who is supposed to love you unconditionally. From that very first moment of humiliation by someone you trust, you step onto your journey of suffering with the potential of surrendering into exquisite grace. While it may not feel like a blessing on the journey, you are indeed blessed to live a life of reaching your full potential of knowing grace."

"When will grace happen?" I asked.

She replied, "When you are ready to receive it."

THE JOURNEY

Healing our relationship with our parents

Did you know that we choose our parents prior to our Soul incarnating into our physical body? I know that it is hard to wrap your mind around that idea. But, truly, our parents do not "create us"; we choose them on the Soul level to be our parents, and then they create our physical vessel. Our parents are forever our most influential teachers. Therefore, whether we have had an easy or stressful life with our parents, it is incredibly vital to heal our relationships with them.

Sri AmmaBhagavan from the Oneness University teaches that the only relationship we are required to heal is the one with our parents. This relationship is the most important relationship of all. Whether or not we heal our relationship with our parents will have a positive or negative impact on all of our other relationships going forward. Please note that we never have to condone our parents' behaviors; we just have to love them in an unconditional manner (acceptance without judgment). In essence, you have to accept that they were doing the best they knew how at the time. This is not always a natural acceptance and requires a commitment to your healing process.

Understanding the theme of my life

I had what would seem to many an easy and simple upbringing. We had a loving family, good friends, and abundant resources. But, hidden behind these trappings were parental perceptions that would lead me to a personal struggle and many opportunities for personal healings. My earliest memory of my struggle with food began when my grandmother told my mother that I was getting chubby. My mother, being the dutiful daughter, listened to her mother and put me on a diet at age seven. This first diet coincided with summer camp. All of the other campers at my dining table could have dessert, but I could not. My counselor told me that my mother said I had to be on a diet. I would watch enviously as the other campers enjoyed their treats. To this day, I can still see them devouring their desserts. I can recall vividly sitting next to the counselor who felt sorry for me. At least I had her empathy.

This public humiliation in front of the other campers was so overwhelming that every day at lunch, I would run out of the dining room in tears. I can see my seven-year-old self slamming open the two screen doors, running out in tears, and with a feeling of nowhere to go. This experience began my journey of developing a poor body image. Yet, there was an even more insidious lifelong pattern starting at that moment. It was the first of what would be 22 times I would experience public humiliation throughout my life. (Yes, I counted them as part of a healing exercise.) These public humiliations (in addition to my self-humiliation by inducing Bulimia) led to a significant and cyclic destructive pattern in my life.

Recognizing the pattern

This theme of humiliation has been present throughout my life. Here is how you know a topic is a theme in your life: You know those times when you are doing just about anything as an adult, and a childhood memory jumps into your mind? Yes, you know those weird thoughts at weird times. Well, those are typically memories from your theme. My theme is humiliation. What is your theme?

Beyond my perpetual humiliation at summer camp, I can remember all the others just as if they happened yesterday. I recall being accused of touching my father's car after he washed it and being punished because my little hands were the size of the handprint, even though I swore I did not do it. I recall being the fourth-grader whose kilted skirt fell off rounding third base during a kickball game at school, and I can still hear the kids laughing at me. Humiliations continued into middle school with getting my period at age nine and not being able to go swimming or sleep over other people's homes because I was embarrassed about my body. I was often humiliated by the adolescent taunting of my mature feminine body. When I was a senior in high school, I saw my boyfriend, who had gone to college, running around with another girl when I went to visit my brother at the same college—all humiliating experiences.

The pattern continued into college when my college love used me to cheat on his current girlfriend, and she caught us together and screamed at me. My first husband would humiliate me by calling me fat—even though I was a size six substitute aerobics teacher. In my first job out of college, I was fired for complaining that a senior corporate partner was sexually harassing me. And on and on into my adult life. Recognizing the themes or patterns in our life is the first step. Working with a professional to review the impact on your life is paramount to breaking the pattern.

Breaking patterns and themes

The pattern of others humiliating me ceased with my second husband, Ori. His role in my life continues to be to love me, unconditionally. Is our life perfect? Of course not, but any humiliation I would feel from him came from his process of victimizing himself and then my feeling the brunt of it as his life partner. This lifelong pattern of humiliation created a deep fear of being humiliated in me. The self-humiliation I felt by purging my food was a defensive move to protect myself from humiliation by others. In other words, if I humiliated myself first, there would be no room for others to humiliate me.

When I came out of corporate America and into the spiritual arts, I added a new level of fear. I became afraid of being not only humiliated but being persecuted as well. By participating in past-life regressions, I have discovered many lifetimes where I have been tortured and killed by non-tolerant religious establishments. In one past-life regression, I recall running through the woods in deep fear. Behind me was an angry mob carrying pitchforks and whatever barbaric weapons they could find. They chased me until they were close enough for one of their weapons to hit me. I passed out from the blow, but I was still alive. Then, they dug a hole and threw me into the pit, still alive. I landed face up, and they covered me with rocks. In essence, I was buried alive.

I first discovered this past-life regression in a healing session with a mentor. Then, further down my spiritual journey, I returned to this past life with the same mentor in another session. The past-life scenario proceeded the same way except that after I was thrown in the pit, I looked up and saw Yeshua kneeling over the hole with his hand out for me to grab before the rocks tumbled onto me. In essence, my Soul left my physical body before the angry mob could finish the job of killing me.

The first time I experienced this past-life regression, I was only ready to see the persecution. The second time I experienced this past life, I could see that the Divine is available to support us in our most significant moment of need. And, for sure, I needed a helping hand to leave that hell on earth. My past-life experience is just one example of the pain and suffering that spiritual women and men have endured due to religious persecution.

I entered this lifetime with an overwhelming fear of humiliation and persecution, and it had stopped me from fully living my true spiritual nature. I've lived within my spiritual nature probably better than most, although not to the extent that the Divine wanted.

The Divine had a different plan for me.

When I dedicated my life to be of Divine Service, I committed to a life of being in the public eye— sharing information about my life and the teachings that the Divine wanted me to share. I thought I was setting myself up for even possibly greater humiliations and persecutions. Yet, I would discover that this perception of persecution of spiritual teachers in this lifetime was inaccurate. I found that because the stakes are so high for humanity's future, the Divine has established that persecution will not be the path for spiritual teachers.

Instead, we are here to help the world heal and live in an enlightened way in the Golden Age/Age of Aquarius. This time is often referred to as the Age of God, meaning the age where we recognize our Oneness with God. Living in Oneness takes a commitment to our healing, a commitment to living the Divine teachings, and following Divine requests, regardless of how humiliating they may appear to be on the surface.

One time at a conference of professional messengers, I attended a comedian's performance. I heard a male voice from the spiritual realm say, "Get up and go to your room."

I replied, "No, I don't want to get up in the middle of this comedian's routine. He will notice me and say something."

The voice persisted, "Get up and go to your room."

My maternal instinct kicked in, and I thought maybe someone was sick or injured, and I had to make a phone call on their behalf. I got up and walked to the back of the jam-packed ballroom.

I was just about to turn the door handle and exit the room when I heard the comedian say into his microphone, "Where are you going, lady? Am I not funny enough for you?"

I started to turn around to respond, but when I heard the hundreds of people laughing at me, I panicked and ran out the door in probably one of the most humiliating moments of my life. When my roommates came back to our room, I was still so humiliated that I could not take my head out from under the sheet and pretended to be asleep.

In retrospect, I have come to understand many aspects of that experience. The first is that I was crazy- scared to go on stage the next day for my scheduled talk about my writing relationship with Yeshua, even in a forum of like-minded people. Being humiliated in front of the same crowd the night before was intended to take care of my self-fulfilling prophecy of humiliation and persecution for speaking my truth the next day. For, I thought, if they all laughed at me the night before, then they would not boo me or throw things at me the next day.

I imagine that sounds a bit farfetched, but I don't think I would have had the courage to go on the stage the next day. All of my past life experiences were yelling at me, "Don't do this; it's too risky." The next day, hours before my presentation, I said, "Yeshua, I am not going to be able to speak today about *Messiah Within*; I am too afraid."

Yeshua responded, "Who are you, Robin, not to do this for me?"

My entire being knew that what he said was true. Yeshua gave me advice on how to calm myself down on stage and, when it was my turn, I spoke for the very first time about releasing my fear of persecution, which I outlined in *Messiah Within*. My message was well-received by the audience, and I then felt a deep sense of pride and accomplishment.

Coming out of the bathroom

The final example of public humiliation described above occurred at least five years before I was ready to stop being my own humiliator and persecutor. As an additional defensive shield, I have kept on twenty pounds of excess weight, which I carry mostly in my belly. It's like an extra impenetrable layer of protection between me and anyone else. No one would get to me with humiliation or persecution as long as I carried my physical "shield." I knew that recovery for me would include surrendering my suffering with public and self-humiliation.

I knew that to stop humiliating myself through binging and purging; I would have to rely on someone else in addition to myself. This person is someone who would never judge me on my addictive nature, and that is my husband, Ori. If I were moving towards a desire to obsessively eat or consider being bulimic, I would share with him that I was heading in that direction, and he lovingly helped me to back away from the edge of taking adverse action. He also finds comfort in food, so at times we can be each other's worst enemies by bringing poor food choices into our home.

Fortunately, we have been able to find a balance between healthy and unhealthy food choices. Nothing is perfect, and we consistently run at about 90 percent healthy and 10 percent unhealthy. This ratio enabled me to learn to eat peacefully and to stay in recovery. When I think back on the bulimia, I must acknowledge that it did serve me. On a neurotic symbolic note, the bulimia kept me safe in my bathroom from anyone who would show up at my door to persecute me or ostracize me. But guess what . . . no one ever showed up. In fact, "coming out of the bathroom" has shown me that the same person who has loved me unconditionally is still waiting in the living room just outside the bathroom to love me, honor me, protect me "till death do us part."

Entering the Zone of Genius

In *The Big Leap* by Gay Hendricks, the author shares that most of us spend our lives in our Zone of Brilliance. Many of us desire to move up into our Zone of Genius, but are stopped by what he calls "upper limit beliefs." When I visualize these upper limit beliefs, I think of a path in the woods that I am walking down (a metaphor for life). When I get down the trail, there is a large rock (my upper limit beliefs) blocking the path to my genius life. What are my choices? I can stand and stare at that rock and do nothing, or I can jump over it and try to get to my "genius life" without removing my upper limit beliefs, or I can deal with my upper limit beliefs and clear the path to my genius life.

I discovered that what kept me out of my Zone of Genius was my deep fear and belief that I would be humiliated if I lived in my Zone of Genius. Of course, that makes sense, since it is a recurring pattern in my life. My pattern persisted publicly and privately until I was ready to see it and heal it and to accept grace from Sophia, the Universal Mother. Please take a moment to take that in.

What if the pattern is so incredibly crucial on your Soul's journey that you know you must hold onto it until you can see the gift of it? You must keep faith that once you know the gift of the pattern, then you are ready to receive the grace required to heal it. In my lifelong pattern of public and private humiliation, I had no idea of the significance of it. When I went through the exercise of pinpointing all of my humiliating experiences, I knew there had to be a bigger picture that I was missing. In other words, I needed to see how humiliation and addiction tied together in my life.

Humiliation leads to self-loathing.

Was I finally ready to believe that I did not have to humiliate and persecute myself to prevent others from doing it to me? What I discovered was that my bulimia was a way of purging a lifetime assault of public and personal humiliation until I was ready to share it in a more public way to help others. I would privately humiliate myself with purging until I was ready to see the incredible humiliation pattern and live all the teachings that Sophia wanted me to share with you. Here is what I have learned about the pattern of humiliation:

- Humiliation leads to self-loathing;

- Self-loathing leads to struggle;

- Struggle leads to suffering;

- Suffering leads to addiction;

- To heal from addiction, you must surrender;

- When you surrender, grace will arrive;

- Within grace, you will have the tools you need to heal your self-loathing;

- In the process of healing, you will return to self-love;

- When self-love is secure, you can recover from addiction.

For you see, until you can love yourself, you cannot heal from addiction. I know that may sound trite or may be hard to hear, but it is true. I faced the continued assault of public and personal humiliation until I was ready to love myself and then, and only then, could I move into recovery.

Become too full of yourself

Here is a story to ponder: When I was releasing *Messiah Within*, I was scared. Yeshua said to me, "Go outside and walk for 45 minutes. I want you to repeat the following: 'I AM the Messiah Within, I am.' The first I AM calls in the God source, and the second 'I am' declares who you are. I walked for 45 minutes and repeated this mantra, breathing in the beautiful evening air.

When I got home, I walked into the living room and shared with Ori what Yeshua had me do. I was so jazzed up to release the book, and Ori replied, "Don't be too full of yourself." You might be thinking that Ori was dismissive of my excitement, but what I have come to know is that Ori is the most important mirror to what I am feeling inside.

In the past, I would have gotten angry and probably did so when that happened. Ori's words triggered in me the realization that I had heard those words before from my father when I had appeared too excited with a personal accomplishment. I have been trying not to be "too full of myself" my whole life. I had been purging my food to make sure that I was not too full of myself or too full of food.

Today, I am very focused on being "too full of myself"—but now with self-pride and healthy food. If I am too full of myself, when my cup runneth over, what is left in the saucer is always enough for the people who need my support. If I can fill myself up with healthy food and loving thoughts about my life, then my light will shine out to all those I meet. I heal others just by sharing my light. I healed myself by knowing that everything I experienced and continue to experience in this lifetime is an integral part of my unique destiny.

Up to now, we have reviewed the psychological and emotional components of addictions. In the next chapter, let's discuss the silent epidemic of bulimia.

"Sophia, it seems like all the research on bulimia points to a desire to lose weight. Do you concur?" I asked.

Sophia replied, "It is so easy to place the blame for eating disorders squarely on the shoulders of a society obsessed with being thin. More likely, bulimia is a way to release all the pain you are feeling from being human.

Clearly, there are physical, psychological, and cultural issues that impact your view of your body. We desire that you move beyond your pain and into a healthy relationship with your vessel."

UNDERSTANDING BULIMIA

Recognizing a silent epidemic

Is binging and purging a silent epidemic that no one is talking about? Logic suggests that if we have an obesity problem, then, conversely, we must <u>not</u> have a binging and purging problem. Wrong! When you are in a cycle of binging and purging, you don't lose weight. You may get fatter because your body will hold onto every calorie it can to prepare for the famine that most certainly comes after the feast.

Binging and purging (feast and famine) creates the exact opposite outcome that people with this affliction are trying to accomplish. How can we stop the madness of this addictive behavior? First, it is essential to understand what this affliction is. I will share the definition as presented by Bulimia.com, and then I will offer more information on Sophia's perspective on this disorder.

> Bulimia nervosa is an eating disorder usually characterized by periods of binging—or excessive overeating—followed by compensatory behavior. People with bulimia have a fear of gaining weight; however, that does not mean all people with bulimia are underweight. Some people with bulimia are overweight or obese and may attempt to use purging to manage their weight or to prevent additional weight gain. Bulimia nervosa is a serious mental illness

that requires intensive treatment. Getting help for your bulimia gives you the best chance to overcome this eating disorder.

According to the National Institute of Mental Health, 1 percent of the adult population in the United States suffers from bulimia at some point in their life. Another 2.8 percent of the population experiences a binge eating disorder without purging. NIMH eating disorder statistics show that women are more likely than men to develop an eating disorder, including bulimia, binge eating disorder, and anorexia. Younger women are more likely to develop this mental health disorder; however, bulimia affects individuals regardless of gender, age, economic status, or lifestyle. All cases of bulimia are equally valid and require treatment such as therapy, medicine, or inpatient treatment.

Bulimia is an addictive behavior.

I often wonder why it took me more than 40 years to try to find a solution to my addiction. I am confident that it's because I was living my journey until it was the perfect time to write this book. Does that help ease the shame and guilt I feel about abusing my body? No, not really, but I can work on that, too, in my healing journey.

Did you notice that Bulimia.com did not say that obsessive-compulsive food disorder or bulimia was an addiction? They called it an eating disorder and a mental health issue. For purposes of giving this silent epidemic its proper attention, I am giving it the same status as other perceived addictions. But remember, the *primary* addiction is to suffering. The other secondary addictions, such as alcoholism, drugs, and bulimia, should also be called addictions. But by focusing on the secondary addictions and not the primary addiction, we are focusing on the symptoms and not the root problem. Because this is the norm in our society, it is worth spending time defining "addiction" as it is currently perceived.

According to the American Psychiatric Association:

> Addiction is a complex condition, a brain disease that is manifested by compulsive substance use despite harmful consequence. People with addiction (severe substance use disorder) have an intense focus on using a certain substance(s), such as alcohol or drugs, to the point that it takes over their life. They keep using alcohol or a drug even when they know it will cause problems. Yet a number of effective treatments are available, and people can recover from addiction and lead normal, productive lives.
>
> People can develop an addiction to alcohol, marijuana, PCP, LSD and other hallucinogens, inhalants, such as, paint thinners and glue, opioid pain killers, such as codeine and oxycodone, heroin, sedatives, hypnotics and anxiolytics (medicines for anxiety such as tranquilizers), cocaine, methamphetamine, and other stimulants and tobacco.

Binging on sugar

If bulimia is a silent epidemic, then the consumption of sugar must also be categorized as an epidemic, not the least of which because sugar is a favorite binging source for bulimics. In an article on Healthline.com, Dr. Alan Greene, a pediatrician who sits on the board of the Institute for Responsible Nutrition, said, "Sugar- sweetened beverages, along with cakes, cookies, and ice cream, are the major offenders, but hidden sources of added sugars are also a concern. What happens is that Americans are having dessert several times a day and don't know it."

Let's take a moment to learn more about the super sugar addicts who have bulimia. As previously noted, 1 percent of the adult population in the United States suffers from bulimia at some point in their life.

That calculates to 3,300,000 people (mostly women) that NIMH knows of. Remember, this is a silent epidemic for which most women do not get help, so the actual number is unknown.

Sophia shared that bulimia is a way of purging the pain that we have experienced in our lives. Most conversations on bulimia points to it being a problem for women. Have men not experienced pain the same way as women? On a societal level, women are held to a higher standard of vanity than men, so this need to be beautiful may be something much more profound for women, something much more ancient.

In an interesting article by Maria McKeown, *Women Through History: Women's Experience Through the Ages*, she reminds us that "In past societies, women were warriors, powerful priestesses, and political leaders. At other times, strict expectations have been placed on women, portraying them as inferior to men. In many parts of the world today, women do not enjoy equal opportunities to earn, participate in politics, or get an education."

While women have been persecuted since the beginning of humanity, I always was curious as to when the most notorious persecution of spiritual women (particularly of those being accused of witchcraft) began.

In McKeown's article, she writes,

> "Women had traditionally been herbal healers, and their wisdom was very valuable in a world without modern medicine. Often, they gave their help to friends and neighbors freely, or in exchange for small items. As the middle ages wore on, men began to muscle in on what had traditionally been the realm of women. Apothecaries, barber-surgeons, alchemists, and doctors began to compete with herbal cures. Eventually, it became illegal to practice medicine at all without having studied at university, and guess what? Medieval universities did not admit women!

> This persecution culminated in accusations of witchcraft and the mass-burnings of women accused of witchcraft in the 1600s. At the same time, the new male doctors had some interesting perspectives to give on women's health. They regarded women as prone to 'hysteria'

(this word comes from the Latin word for womb), and 'lunacy' (they linked madness to the phases of the moon, and by extension to the female menstrual cycle). Their diagrams of conception showed women as passive empty vessels that merely hosted the male seed. It wasn't until the 1900s that medical science recognized that women provide 50 percent of DNA in the creation of a baby!"

Bulimia as self-punishment

Could this also represent a common thread that pertains to all women with bulimia? Is bulimia a global form of self-punishment derived from thousands of years of religious persecution? The following is a promise that I have shared many times in coaching sessions with spiritual women. "It never ended well before." says the Divine to all spiritual women. "But in this lifetime, it will end well," ensures the Divine.

Throughout history, spiritual women have endured deep suffering and relentless persecution, supposedly in the name of the Divine. In this lifetime, spiritual women have a deep knowing that the true Divine co-creates our lives with us and, therefore, it is possible have the lives we most desire.

It will end well.

But first, we must heal our collective belief that suffering and persecution are required today, just like this belief persisted for thousands of years. Indeed, bulimia is the act of being the victim AND the persecutor in your life. Overeating and then purging is just one way to be the victim and the persecutor of your life. If you are fortunate to live in a country where you are not being persecuted, then thank goodness! However, many women in this world still live under the tyranny of this kind of persecution. Sometimes when I am sharing a channeled message that is particularly profound, I say to myself, "Off with your head!" as a reminder of how blessed I am to be here in the 21st century and not in an earlier century.

I believe that it is almost guaranteed that if you are a deeply spiritual woman reading this book, then you have lost past lives for your beliefs. Perhaps my own experience has been so extreme precisely so that I may bring this ancient pain to light and give spiritual women a voice with which to express the incredible suffering that we have endured since the beginning of time. In "remission," it is easy for me to "remember my mission."

I have purged enough pain for this lifetime and all of my past lifetimes as a spiritual messenger who was condemned to torture and death by societies that were not ready to live their spiritual nature. Thank goodness it will end well in this lifetime and that I have the freedom to share my story with you. The message from the Divine (that it will end well for all of us) should enable you to live the life that truly speaks to your own heart. Be bold, be brave, and serve to your heart's content!

So many of us are held back by our fears and our need to be perfect. In Chapter Five, let's discuss how perfectionism can derail our real spiritual mission.

"Sophia, there is so much pressure for every little girl or boy to be perfect in the eyes of their parents. Isn't that a lot to ask for?" I asked.

Sophia replied, "First of all, you were born perfect, and you are perfect now in the eyes of the Divine. Other questions you might want to ask are why does society have a different view on what perfection is and why is it so unattainable, and why does it matter so much?

In other words, why does humanity look for perfection on the outside versus on the inside? My last, but most important question to humanity is, "Why are you all so afraid of your Divine perfection?"

THE PERFECT DAUGHTER

What would others think?

My father, George, was a professional man. Everything we did was measured as to whether it would embarrass my father in his capacity as a professional man. I can remember hearing, "You are the daughter of a professional man; act accordingly." What did that mean to a teenager? I knew that I had to live up to a standard, but I was not sure what that meant to someone like me who was wild and free. My father held high standards for his children, and it always seemed like he was frustrated with us. My dad was a respected dentist, a pillar of the community, and yet he seemed to hold expectations for his children, perhaps based on the hopes that his parents had for him.

My mother, Mona, played the traditional stay at home role while her children were young. To keep peace in the house, she would do her best to protect us from my father's strict standards. Sometimes that meant helping us too much with our homework or doing chores for us. She intended to keep the peace but may have created an enabling atmosphere for her children. My mom was involved in philanthropic events and a pillar of the community. When I was in middle school, my mom went to work, and she became a successful real estate broker. Like my father, she seemed to hold expectations for her children, perhaps based on the hopes that her parents had for her.

My two loving parents focused on perfection, each in their way. My dad's focus was on how we would look to the outside world; "what would other people think?" My mom's attention was on keeping us well-behaved and making sure that we presented well to the outside world; "what would other people think?" In an article by Mel Schwartz, "The Problem with Perfection," he writes:

> The desire to be perfect burdens many people and ironically dooms them to unhappiness. Humans were never intended to be perfect. That's part of the definition of being human. Consider the expression, "I'm just human." We need to remind ourselves the goal isn't to emulate a machine, but to embrace the imperfection of being human. We forget that as humans, we're part of nature, as well. As such, we would benefit if we came into acceptance of the natural state of life, which by the way happens to be imperfect. Usually, we strive toward being perfect to compensate for a sense of inadequacy. People who want to be perfect usually have an exaggerated sense of their shortcomings. They typically received messages earlier in life that they weren't good enough. Individuals who seek perfection are acutely sensitive to the judgments of others. In fact, these judgments are most often imagined. Everyone has an opinion, and elevating someone else's opinion to the status of being a judge is really silly. After all, someone else can't really judge you unless you confer upon him or her, the power of being a judge.

Yikes, did I confer the power of being a judge onto my parents? Of course, I did! I was a child, then a teenager, then a young adult, then a middle-aged adult, and it wasn't until recently that I removed them from the judge's bench. This is an important concept worth repeating: we chose our parents before we incarnated into this lifetime. I chose the "perfect" parents, who would teach me to strive for perfection with a healthy dose of feelings of unworthiness.

Doing the best they could

When I began my spiritual journey, I was sent to the Oneness University in Chennai, India, to heal my inner child. We were sitting in complete darkness, reviewing our childhood. In that session, my parents appeared to me energetically and sat with me. They were young, and I remember hearing them say, "We did the very best we knew how to do based on who we were at that moment in time."

I have come to understand what that means. There were moments raising my children when I would say or do something that I felt was harmful, and I would say to myself, "Well, there's a moment for my children to review on the therapist's couch!" For sure, our parents were not perfect, as we are not perfect as parents, just as nobody is perfect in this human game called Life. Yet, Sophia said that we are perfect. How do we reconcile this? We are indeed perfect as Divine beings and most likely perfect as human beings, but we just don't cut ourselves enough slack. When I think about my journey to *divine perfection*, I am transported back to when I started purging my food.

Maintaining a perfect image

Like many of us who grew up in the 1970s, I liked to party my brains out. My parents would go out on a Saturday night, and one of my brothers and I would have a party in the house. My other brother would provide the weed, and everyone else would bring food. We would get incredibly high, and then we would pig-out on food—all the while laughing hysterically. At some point, I would make my way to the bathroom. I came to understand that if I made myself throw up, not only would I not get fat, but I would also come down from my high in time to be in front of my parents. By the time they arrived home, the house was picked up, our friends were gone, and I was back to being the perfect daughter of a professional man.

My father passed away many years ago, and I have been fortunate to connect with him as needed through my spiritual abilities and the abilities of my spiritual colleagues. In a recent session with a medium, my father returned to tell me, "It is still important to me that you are perfect." At first, I took this as *"Really, Dad? Still busting me?"* but then I realized that in the spiritual realm, he must have the same definition as Sophia. Therefore, I can declare I AM perfect, Dad!

My mother is my greatest teacher.

Finding peace with my mother around body image took a bit more work. She is a constant reminder of my relationship with food. She would talk to me daily about her weight or the weight of others if I allowed it. We have an agreement that the topic of weight is off-limits, but my mom does not comply. Ironically, she does not comply by complimenting me that I look thinner.

I believe in her heart; she thinks this is what I want to hear her tell me. Perhaps I do, but somewhere along the line, it triggered my sense of not being good enough. For you see, each person in our lives is a mirror to our self; each is here to teach us something. I have had a lot to learn about my bulimia from my mom.

I was on a radio show, and my mother saw a picture of me from that show and said, "I wanted to tell you, your face looked thinner." What I was hoping for was validation for my accomplishment. I had to look for it from myself. In her way, perhaps my mom was validating my accomplishment.

When I arrive at her home in Florida, the first thing she says is, "You look thinner." I would be happier with *"you look healthy"* or *"you look wonderful."* But maybe, from her perspective, that's what she means.

On one visit to Florida, I knew that I had to have a serious conversation with my mom about writing this book. The talk would not be easy, and I would have to remember that I chose her to be my mom because my Soul knew that she would play her part in my bulimia play with a "Tony Award-winning" performance. She would hold the energy of the bulimia with me until I was ready to write this book.

The bulimia play is closed.

As of the last day in Florida, I still had not had a conversation about the book with my mom. With two hours to go before leaving, I was feeling a sense of relief for not having talked with her about it when my mom said, "You know, Rob, I never throw up my food." I spun around in my chair, ready to react, but before I could, something extraordinary happened.

I felt my higher self, or my Soul, come out of my body and stand next to my chair. When I responded to her, I could feel the words coming out of my mouth, but my higher consciousness was observing the interaction.

I replied, "Good for you. I have probably thrown up thousands of times over 40 years." She then said, "I am sorry to hear that. You know, Robin, I am never going to change."

My higher self looked down at me and said, "Did you hear her, Robin? She is never going to change."

From that moment on, I decided that I would stop trying to make her change for me to feel safe from her words about my weight. I had been waiting for my mom to change so that I could take control over my own body. Now, I no longer had to hold onto my suffering. I finally realized that if I don't view her as a tormentor, then I don't have to be afraid of her words. From that moment on, I was no longer anxious about seeing my mom or worried about what she would say.

Well, maybe a little bit. After all, it has been a dynamic between us for more than 50 years. Other than our body image dance, I have had an excellent relationship with my mom. She is kind, funny, and loves me to the moon and back. We spend most of our time in other interesting conversations about our family, friends, and the state of the world. Now, I am excited to be with my mom without the fear of feeling humiliated. When she says, I look thinner; I will know that she is saying I love you.

Moving from fear and humiliation to love and light is the path I have chosen, but it doesn't come without challenges. Let's explore what it means to be on the spiritual path in Chapter Six.

Sophia's Insights for Chapter Six

"Sophia, why is it so hard for people to find their way onto the spiritual path?" I asked.

Sophia replied, "Quite simply, Robin, they are afraid. When in fear, they cannot see the light that guides them to a joyous life. Fear is so debilitating, and it is promoted by all of the systems on your planet: religion, politics, health, entertainment, and education.

If all you are taught is fear, then how can you live from love? The spiritual path is for brave Souls who choose to live as love and not allow the fear to consume them. Will spiritual seekers know fear and pain?

Of course, they welcome it, because you must go through the pain and fear of the past to get to the light and love of the present. From the light-filled present, you can move forward to a magnificent future."

CHAPTER SIX

THE PATH TO SPIRIT

Last-minute Soul substitution

When I was growing up, I would hear my Mom tell a story that right before my birth, she changed my name from Roberta to Robin. Later in life on my spiritual journey, I was told that the Soul energy in my physical vessel replaced the Soul energy that was initially in my body right before my birth. I have always found that to be an interesting correlation between the new Soul energy and my new name. Who was this new Soul energy that needed to come into this body?

It was a Soul energy that would be able to sustain a life of humiliation and self-persecution to be able to write a book to help others to heal. In my work with clients, I often find that we are here to teach what we most needed to learn. When my clients hear that their lives have been a training ground for filling their Soul's destiny, they are often relieved because all the good, the bad, and the ugly experiences in their lives were all worth it.

First contact from Spirit

My most vivid memory of being spiritual was when I was in my first job in public accounting. I was working on a Saturday in the middle of tax season. I stood up in the middle of the bullpen (a room of newbie accountants) and announced, "I have to go to Manhattan now." I called my family and told them to meet me at my grandmother's room in the hospital. I grabbed my purse and ran to catch a train. I entered my grandmother's room and sat quietly by her bed. My family began to arrive, and we waited.

I was holding my grandmother's hand, and she said to me, "Don't look at them, they are not here for you." I promised I would not look, but she did not believe me.

She placed her hands over my eyes. I started to laugh and said, "I promise I won't look."

I have wondered if my grandmother knew of my spiritual gifts since it seemed she wanted to make sure I did not leave with the assembly of loved ones and angels who were ready to take her home. She quietly took her last breath and transitioned to the non-physical. When it was time to leave, my family quietly made a joke and said, "When you get a message to come to see me urgently, don't come." This was my introduction to communicating with another being's Soul energy. The next time would be right before my father's passing.

"Get my daughter on the phone."

That day began as a typical day in corporate America in the 1990s except with one unique exception—my dear friend was selling jewelry in the lobby of my office building. She never sold one piece of jewelry, and we were talking at lunch, thinking this was a waste of time. And then I felt this deep knowing to go back up to the phone at my desk. We did not have cell phones at the time, so we had actually to go to a landline phone. When I arrived at my office, my desk phone was ringing. I answered the phone, and it was my mom telling me that she and my brother were on their way from New Jersey to Philadelphia because my father was dying.

I called Ori and said, "I want to call my father, but I am afraid." Ori replied, "What do you have to lose, Robin? Make the call."

I called my father's hospital room, and a nurse picked up the phone. I said, "This is Dr. Handler's daughter, Robin. May I please speak to my father?"

She replied, "Oh my goodness, all your father keeps repeating is, "Get my daughter on the phone, get my daughter on the phone."

She gave the phone to my dad, and I said, "dad, please don't worry about mom, we will always take care of her. I love you very much."

With the message received, my father passed away. My dear friend (who was from New Jersey) drove me back to New Jersey to be with my mother.

Living as the Divine

These two experiences with two important loved ones began a path of learning that would take me to who I have become today: a profoundly spiritual person committed to living as the Divine on this earth plane. How does an everyday working mom become a Divine Emissary? It takes a lot of commitment and resources. The resources come in many forms, from funds to study with extraordinary teachers to opening myself to create an exceptional network of like-minded people with whom to share the journey. Over the years, I thought that I had to exclude some oppositional and toxic people from my life. I came to realize that all I needed to do was stand firm in my convictions and live the life that was unfolding in front of me. My family and friends would choose to accept me for who I had become, or they would leave.

The spiritual path would unfold precisely as my Soul intended before this incarnation in my physical body. In my work with clients on their Soul Plan—in-depth knowledge of what their Soul's destiny is— they are always pleasantly surprised to hear and see that their life has been unfolding perfectly. If you can relax into this knowing, your life becomes a magical, mystical tour of mind-blowing events. Does this surprise you? If you commit to fulfilling your Soul's destiny, then all of these experiences must occur. It is part of the plan! My path of profound spiritual learning and healing has included opportunities to travel to other countries and to achieve certifications in healing modalities. I have had to heal traumas from this and past lives. These encounters were never easy but required me to move forward to my destiny. This phase of study and healing on the spiritual path is called "Mastery."

Mastery is a stage of spiritual development where you remain in the struggle until you are ready to move forward into the stages of Service and Leadership. The stage of Mastery is defined as the endless pursuit of spiritual knowledge and inner healing work. We get stuck here because we are not ready to release our struggle and surrender. Once we surrender, we can receive the gift of knowing the actual reason behind the struggle and then receive the grace to resolve the struggle. When you get stuck in the Mastery phase, you limit what is coming next. There is much more available to you on your spiritual journey beyond study and healing. If you are here on the spiritual journey, you are here to serve and lead others in their lives, defined as Service and Leadership on the spiritual journey.

The spiritual journey is unfolding.

There is nothing one can do to push it along. You may get a hint about a future knowing or healing that is coming, but it will not fully manifest until Divine Timing occurs. When the Divine realm is sharing a message with me, I have learned to discern if it is for the present moment or the future. At first, I had no expertise with spiritual discernment, meaning that I would jump and do whatever I was told to do by Spirit at that moment in time. Yes, I was blessed to hear the message, but did that mean I should immediately focus my attention on what was shared in the message?

Sometimes the message I received was intended for my current spiritual growth. And other times, it was a message meant for my future. As an example, I received the request from Sophia to write this book two years before I was ready to begin. I had not lived all of the experiences that would lead to the knowledge I share in this book. I had to trust that Divine Timing would show me the right time to start.

And yet, I started anyway because, after all, Sophia requested it. What resulted was a book on recovery from addiction written prematurely, while I was in active addiction. I would never achieve the ending or, more importantly, the impact that I was trying to make. I decided to put the book manuscript down and wait for the right time to begin again. In other words, I was waiting to be in recovery so I could share a solution that works. In my earlier haste to finish, I tried to hire a ghostwriter, and that did not work because *she* was not requested to write this book, *I* was. And then, the Divine Timing unfolded, and now here I am with the properly finished work.

Divine Timing rules the clock.

The concept of Divine Timing adds a layer of complexity because we live according to linear time on the earth plane, and there is no concept of time in the non-physical world. How can the two be reconciled? Quite simply, you cannot do what Spirit is suggesting as a solution if you have yet to live the problem they are helping you to resolve.

My first encounter with Divine Timing happened when I was writing *Messiah Within*. I was stuck on how to get going on writing this book (In other words, I had no idea what to write.). I was sitting at my Grandmother's desk in my sacred family home, and Yeshua came to me. He said, "How about if I tell you the 12 Steps to becoming your Messiah Within?"

I replied, "That would be great!"

So, He began, "Step 1 is…" all the way to "Step 12 is …"

I read them to myself and realized that I had lived the first ten over the prior eight years, and I had not yet lived the last two steps. When would steps 11 and 12 happen? I had no clue, but I knew I had to be exceptionally patient.

At times, I thought I was living Step 11 or Step 12, but it wasn't feeling quite right. How would I come to know what were the real Steps 11 and 12? Quite simply, the life experience that was required to learn the lesson of Steps 11 and 12 came with the same spiritual and life-altering experiences that had ushered the previous ten steps into my life. When Step 11 arrived, there was no question that was it. The same happened for Step 12—it was almost like getting hit over the head with a spiritual 2 x 4!

The spiritual journey is the most exciting and the most challenging journey of your life. The more committed you are, the harder it is because you have to heal your wounds of the past. However, by committing to this level of mastery—both in self-healing and study—you can access your Divine Right to a life filled with abundant blessings.

As you prepare to be of Divine service, part of your work is to heal your emotional wounds. Chapter Seven talks more about this and my path to alleviating long-standing suffering.

"Sophia, what are the qualifications you look for in someone who is on their way to be of Divine service?"

Sophia laughed. "First of all, Robin, there is no job interview required. A person becomes of Divine service when they are genuinely inspired to share what they have learned on their spiritual journey.

Most often, teachers of spiritual information have been deeply wounded themselves, and they have committed to healing themselves.

When they become genuinely grateful for the grace bestowed upon them by knowing how to heal their pain and suffering, they want to share that with others.

Divine service can be a simple smile to a stranger or writing a book on behalf of the Divine realm. It all serves."

CHOOSING TO HEAL AND SERVE

Authenticity is Key

I began my career in the spiritual arts as a spiritual promoter by creating spiritual events for other spiritual teachers and distributing spiritual cinema. I pursued that path until I was asked by Yeshua to become an author and a teacher. While I reluctantly did what I was asked, I didn't feel like I was ready to truly serve the Divine until now, by writing this book. My dilemma was that I was being asked to be a spiritual author and teacher at a time when I felt like I was not spiritually authentic. This feeling of spiritual inauthenticity or, in other words, being an addict and being a spiritual teacher, felt like two polar extremes.

Where was the authentic Robin? Where was the Robin who believed in Oneness? Where was the Robin who knew that she is the Creator of her own life and that she must live a process of deep emotional clearing if she is ever going to stand proudly in the teachings she had received? She was busy overeating and purging and teaching spirituality. She was the model of the wounded healer.

The Wounded Healer

The wounded healer in astrology and metaphysics was a centaur known as Chiron. In an article by James Robinson (Elephant Journal), the author shares that, "Although Chiron was the god of healing, he could not heal himself. He was forced to live with incredible pain until he chose to give up his immortality. Ultimately, Chiron represents something we all carry in our subconscious mind. He is that which will kill us if we don't heal it— our deepest wounds, our fatal flaws. Again, it represents our deepest wounds that, when overcome, become our biggest strengths."

Robinson shares that there are certain personality traits wounded healers carry:

- We tend to take things more personally than others. It is this very sensitivity that causes us such deep pain that helps us understand others' suffering.

- We cause our suffering. Until we learn to take responsibility for our wounds, we cannot heal our wounds and take responsibility for our recovery.

- We have to give something up. When we let go of preconceived notions about what is required for success, the struggling stops, as well as the pain.

- We have to learn to shrug it off. We mustn't value what others think of us over how we value ourselves.

Not valuing others over ourselves is especially crucial for addicts.

In his article, Robinson explains how the Wounded Warrior and the addict are connected. "Chiron was more highly evolved than other centaurs. Most centaurs, beings that were half-man, half-horse, were concerned only with earthly pleasures, especially sex and mind/mood-altering drugs. Chiron was only interested in healing and higher planes of being. Ironically, Chiron was attacked by others of his kind when he opened a jar of wine to serve to Hercules. The others' addiction to pleasure forced them to attack, and it was a mindless and fatal decision for most of them."

Robinson reminds us in this article that we must be careful about our addictions and attachments to worldly pleasures as they can set us up for attacks not only by strangers but by those we love. Being able to withstand criticism or humiliation is a common wound that most wounded healers must heal. As wounded healers heal, they rise to their true I AM and don't care what others think of them.

Don't go back to sleep!

When we think of a spiritual teacher, we often think of someone who is a grounded, profoundly connected person who honors their vessel, does all of their healing work, studies spirituality consistently, and connects to the Divine through meditation. Yet, in reality, no spiritual teacher can be all of those attributes, all the time.

This poem by Rumi explains the path of the spiritual teacher:

> The breezes at dawn have secrets to tell you Don't go
> back to sleep!
>
> You must ask for what you really want.
>
> Don't go back to sleep!
>
> People are going back and forth
>
> Across the doorsill where the two worlds touch,
>
> The door is round and open.
>
> Don't go back to sleep!

I love this poem because staying in our Divine nature is a moment by moment process. "Don't go back to sleep," symbolizes how easy it can be to live unaware or aware. The choice is present at each moment. As the poem implies, spiritual teachers live in two worlds: the everyday earth plane and the spiritual realm that is beyond our five senses. Our work is to stay awake to the Divine possibilities while still being grounded in the physical world.

Becoming of Divine service

The most important responsibility of the spiritual teacher, author, practitioner, or counselor is to keep moving forward in their spiritual growth, even if it is only one step at a time. This personal path of growth and healing gives you the exact knowledge that you need to help another. I learned that I only needed to be one step ahead of my clients/students because if I was too far ahead of them, how could I reach for their hand to guide them when they needed help?

When we are asked to be of Divine service, there is an expectation from others and ourselves that we behave in a certain way, and we think that how others perceive us is paramount. Is that true, or are those parental tapes playing in our heads around being perfect? Sophia reminds us that we are perfect just as we are. If that is true, then a spiritual teacher who might occasionally respond to adversity by giving someone "the finger" is perfect, too!

Leonard Cohen wrote, "There is a crack in everything, that is how the light gets in." In essence, we must break open our shields of protection and allow the Divine light to come shining in. When Yeshua asked me to become a Divine Emissary, it meant that I needed to do whatever was needed to heal my wounded messenger persona. Did being a wounded healer stop me from following Yeshua's request or Sophia's request? Absolutely not!

In retrospect, my working on their assignments to share my spiritual journey was like the sincerest form of therapy. To write my books, I had to live simultaneously in the present moment while digging deeply into my past.

Before completing *Messiah Within*, a publicist asked me, "What are your future plans for the book?" I just laughed and said, "I can't go to the future just yet. It's hard enough being in the past and the present at the same time."

Write your story

Writing about one's own lifelong journey/spiritual journey is an incredibly brave act that I highly recommend to everyone. Do you have to publish it? Of course not, but what you will discover about yourself and the connections to family, friends, and the Divine will be extraordinary. If you allow the words to flow from your heart, you will learn more about yourself than from any other form of self-discovery.

What I discovered in my first two books was that I could unveil the teachings that were intended for me to learn on my life journey so that I could share them with others. Yet, they were all written from the place of my wounded messenger. Yes, my words were real, and yes, those were my experiences, and I am proud of them.

However, from an energetic standpoint, I was unable to put the energy behind the books to make them soar into the world to reach as many readers as I could. To be honest, I was afraid of my books. Because I wrote these books in addiction, I was somewhat ashamed of myself; yet, there was an interesting and somewhat contradictory phenomenon taking place with my Soul.

Grounding my Soul in my body

Being in active addiction, I would not allow my Soul energy to inhabit the body that I was victimizing— which happened to be my body. I would do all of my spiritual work with my Soul out in the field of my higher self. What I mean by the sentence above is that our Soul is very expansive (way beyond our body), and only those aspects of our Soul that we need for this lifetime are within our body. Until I could trust myself not to persecute myself, my Soul aspects required for this lifetime could not stay in my body. The only way I could return my Soul to my own body was to dive deeply into my woundedness.

I did this work by collaborating with my human and my etheric support teams. I entrusted my journey to members of my spiritual healing tribe who had previously lived the examined life journey before me. In these women, I found the perfect combination of integrative medicine and energy healing shared in the light of profound wisdom, radical truthfulness, and Oneness.

By combining my deep desire to heal my woundedness with my deep connection to the Divine, I was able to come into remission from my addiction. I must also thank my loving husband, my children, and my dog, Hailey, who all provided me with unconditional love in the safest container of family. I also had to shift some friendships to a different level of connection, and new amazing friends have entered my life.

Making peace with my body

There is an anonymous quote in social media that I always stop to read: *"I said to my body softly, 'I want to be your friend. It took a long breath and replied, 'I have been waiting my whole life for this."* I resolve to make peace with my body finally. Does that mean that I won't overeat? I know that I will—I love food too much. But by being out of the cycle of binging and purging, I am more conscious of what I am eating.

Therefore, by committing to healing my physical, mental, spiritual, and emotional health all at the same time, remission was possible. Now, in remission, my Soul is grounded in my physical body, and I am whole and powerful. And from this place of wholeness, I am writing this book.

No more hiding!

At lunch one day, a dear friend shared a Divine message with me, she said, "There is no one above you." A simple message, and yet my ego started to freak out. It always starts to freak out when I am reminded of my spiritual power. No matter where my spiritual path has taken me with the blessing of enlightened teachers and a true knowing of Oneness, I still get scared of my power. There is a fear deep inside me that if I genuinely share the powerful teachings that live inside me, I will be persecuted. Who am I to not share these teachings that could help so many others heal from addiction? In our lives, we can choose to serve ourselves or serve others or serve the Divine. In essence, all three are the same because we are One. The gift of serving from the place of our healed woundedness is a profound gift of grace to others.

To truly teach what you most came here to learn means you must be willing to expose yourself in your most vulnerable state. There is no more hiding. You must reveal and heal your deepest wounds and learn to serve your Soul. This means surrounding yourself with loving beings of light, both human and etheric. It also means you have to become an open book and know that all of your experiences are intended to help others move through their journey. My work consists of coaching clients who arrive ready to hear the wisdom that I have gathered along my life journey. By healing my wounds, I set off a resonance that attracts others who are serious about healing their wounds and living a life of Divine freedom.

Become the spiritual hero of your own life. Heal your wounds, share your knowledge by teaching others how to thrive. Your Soul fulfills its mission in your personal, professional, and community life. Therefore, you do not have to become a professional healer necessarily—just share how you have healed with others who need to hear what you have to say, and when you do, and you will be fulfilling your Divine service.

Let's take a closer look at what leads people to rely on addictive substances or behaviors to make themselves feel better, and how to find that feeling from within.

"Sophia, is there a cure for addiction?" I asked.

Sophia gently laughed and said, "Is that not the reason for this book, Robin? However, I do understand your confusion because the common belief is that there is not a cure for addiction; therefore, you can never be in remission, like with other diseases.

The cure for addiction is a genuine change in lifestyle that is achieved by a deep connection to your Divine nature, a healthy living environment, a commitment to your wellness, and healing of the negative core beliefs that made addiction seem like the solution to your problems.

Because the cure is esoteric and holistic in nature, society is not quite ready to buy into our solution. With the rise in addiction, eyes will be opened to new approaches. That we know for sure."

MINDSET AND ENVIRONMENT

Recovery, remission, cure

A **cure** is a substance or procedure that ends a medical condition, a medication, a surgical operation, a change in lifestyle, or even a philosophical mindset that helps end a person's sufferings and brings them into the state of being healed or cured. This definition clearly states that what is required is a combination of solutions that impact mind, body, spirit, and emotion.

Because the terms recovery, remission, and cure define the path to wellness, let's take a moment to review Merriam-Webster's definition of recovery, remission, and cure. According to Merriam-Webster, the definition of **recovery** is the process of combating a disorder (such as alcoholism). The definition of **remission** is to abate symptoms (as of a disease) for a period of time. The definition of **cure** is to restore to health, soundness, or normality, to bring about recovery from a disease.

Why no perceived cure for addiction?

Yet, in the traditional Alcoholics Anonymous 12-Step Program, addicts are reminded that they are never cured of addiction. According to www.drugabuse.gov, like other chronic diseases such as heart disease or asthma, treatment for drug addiction usually isn't a cure. However, addiction can be managed successfully. Treatment enables people to counteract addiction's disruptive effects on their brain and behavior and regain control of their lives.

As I typed the information above, I felt a sense of anger. I could hear myself asking, "Why can't we do better than that? Why can't we get out of the 'trying to control our lives' stage to living in full remission? Why can't we be cured of addiction? My research reveals that the experts think you cannot cure addiction because you cannot control the craving. Therefore, you can implement all the steps to get clean and stay clean, but because you cannot clear all the cravings, you are always at risk of falling out of recovery.

Managing cravings is vital

According to Narconon, "A drug craving for an addictive substance is sharper, stronger and much more intense. An addicted person experiencing drug cravings will feel like life itself is dependent on getting and consuming whatever substance is causing those cravings." I certainly know of and have experienced this powerful, driving feeling in my own life. When my obsessive food compulsion would take over, it was like another being was living inside my body. My Soul watched this being take over my body as it became a scavenger for food as if I was never going to eat again.

An example of this occurred one Saturday night when I ordered delivery of an eggplant parmesan dinner. It was a large serving that came with what seemed like a half-pound of pasta. I ate about one-third of the eggplant parmesan and a cup of the pasta. Working diligently to eat a sensible portion, when I felt myself starting to lose control, I threw the rest in the garbage. I know that it was a waste of food and money, but I had to do it. Of course, I was bummed the next day when I had no leftovers.

Even though I had thrown two-thirds of a meal, I decided I wanted dessert. I was alone, and no one was home, I could eat whatever I wanted. So, I ordered delivery of this giant (and I mean **giant**) chocolate chip cookie with ice cream and hot fudge. I was both excited and disappointed in myself while awaiting its arrival. When the dessert arrived, I sat down in front of the TV to enjoy the sweet and declared, "I promise I will only have a few bites." Then the craziest thing happened, my jaw locked! I could not open my mouth to eat the cookie.

Was my body doing an intervention? Perhaps my vessel did not trust me to take just a few bites. I could only drink the melted vanilla ice cream through my partially opened mouth and had to throw out the cookie. Yes, more wasted food and money, but I had to listen to my body and my Soul. In essence, this is no different than an alcoholic spilling his alcohol down the drain or a smoker tossing her cigarettes in the trash. We have to do whatever is required at the moment to quell the cravings.

When I think about that evening, beyond the magical intervention by my body, I wonder why I ordered all of that food in the first place. I know that I was feeling lonely because my husband was away, and I had no other plans or people to hang out with. In my loneliness, I turned to my constant companion over my lifetime: food. What if I had just stayed with the feeling of loneliness, watching it come and go in my energetic field, instead of reacting to the loneliness and ordering lots of food? Indeed, that would have been less wasteful and expensive, but that is not what I was ready to experience that night. Feeding our food addiction is so easy because there is 24-hour access to food. All I can do is continue to raise my awareness, be connected to my body, and experience life from there.

Recognize your loneliness

One of the essential pieces of advice that I received as I began my recovery was that I should go to Weight Watchers, now more familiarly known as "WW." In their meetings, members share their eating experiences from week to week. It is the job of the WW leader to help the members shift their mindset to a combined one of weight loss and wellness. Beyond that, WW provides compulsive eaters with a supportive group environment. In researching loneliness in recovery, I discovered that it was a specific topic.

According to Anaheim Lighthouse Rehab Center, "Loneliness is a dangerous emotion for people in sobriety, especially for those in early sobriety. It is, therefore, essential that the individual begins forming friendships. A network of clean and sober friends can not only help with loneliness, but they will also be a good resource for support and advice." Their website gives solid advice on how to control the dangerous emotion of loneliness, which I paraphrase here:

1. **The Need for New Friends in Recovery:** It is essential to make new clean and sober friends and to say goodbye to some old friendships to have a successful recovery. The key is not to become lonely because loneliness can lead you back to your addictive nature.

2. **The Need for Social Support:** Human beings are social animals, and they depend on a network of other humans to provide support functions. A sober social group offers *emotional support*, physical assistance, and can be a good source of information.

3. **Importance of Friendship in Early Recovery:** Friendship and socialization are especially vital because when you first become sober, you can feel vulnerable, lonely, and bored. Hanging out with others who have been successfully clean can become a source of inspiration.

4. **Loneliness as a Relapse Trigger:** A relapse trigger is a feeling or event that increases the chances an individual will return to active addiction. Therefore, it is essential to stay connected and avoid loneliness.

5. **How to Make Friends in Recovery:** Addicts often struggle with low self-esteem, and they tend to carry this with them into recovery. This lack of self-confidence can be uncomfortable around new people. By joining a base group, they will automatically get to meet a new bunch of people with at least one shared common interest.

Why not me?

Often when I was in active addiction, I would look longingly at friends in long-term recovery and wonder how they did it. While in addiction, I would often ask myself, "Why can that person move into recovery and remission, and I am finding it so difficult?" The answer must be in a change of lifestyle and a shift in mindset. As previously defined, a cure is a change in lifestyle or even a philosophical mindset that helps end a person's sufferings; or the state of being healed or cured.

Albert Einstein said, "We cannot solve our problems with the same thoughts that we used when we created them." We must not only shift our mindset, but we must create a new environment that does not encourage our addictive nature. For example, when I am focused on my health and wellness, I am not thinking obsessive thoughts about "pigging out." When I couple that with not keeping a lot of unhealthy snacks in the house (that is, changing my environment) and limiting the frequency with which I go out to eat, then I am less likely to experience obsessive-compulsive eating.

Even now, any obsessive-compulsive food behavior while eating in a social setting triggers a desire to purge, but I am committed not to do so. Also, feeling like crap from eating crappy food is a far better alternative to purging. The key for me is to stay focused on my health and wellness and eat sensibly. This conversation is my constant companion in my head, all day, every day. But this is the only way I know to manage the cravings, which I have to admit, remain present every day, too. Focusing on my health and wellness equals changing my mindset. Filling my pantry and refrigerator with healthy food and choosing sensibly at restaurants equals changing my environment.

Mindset in recovery

According to Desert Cove Recovery, there are two types of mindsets in addiction. The following information from their website provides excellent examples of the two mindsets.

The first, less desirable mindset is a fixed mindset, and the second, more desirable, is a growth mindset.

Fixed Mindset:

1. *You believe that some people are better equipped to handle life's problems than others.*
2. *You also think that you can't do anything to break free from addiction or change your life.*
3. *You feel stuck when you're in a fixed mindset.*

Growth Mindset:

1. *You can gain almost any skill you want if you have a growth mindset, and nothing can stand in your way.*
2. *You realize that you can solve almost any problem that presents itself with creative ways to reach your desired outcome.*
3. *You will find the motivation and inspiration needed to leave your addiction behind.*

Change your environment.

Another critical part of addiction recovery is changing your environment. In an article by Recovery Ranch, the crucial factor in moving into remission from addiction is to change your environment. Their article states that "What we know now about behaviors is that when they are frequent and that when they repeatedly occur in the same environment, our brains go on autopilot when performing those behaviors. Think about how much your mind can wander as you drive to work, and yet you still get there. You perform the same behaviors so often in the environment of your car and route to work that you can do it without thinking about it."

The article also clearly states that the same works for addiction. To be successful in your recovery, you must create an environment that enables you to be successful. For example, if you are trying to stop eating sugar, eat somewhere new. Instead of reaching for a sugary treat, drink a glass of water or eat an apple. If you want to change a behavior, it is essential to think about how you can alter your environment.

I firmly believe that it is time to stop saying there is no cure for addiction. It's true that to date, we know of no surgery or medical procedure that will cure addiction. We do know, however, that a shift of mindset and change of environment is a significant part of finding one's cure for addiction.

In the next chapter, I will share my journey to remission from addiction in greater detail, highlighting the mind, body, spiritual, and emotional approach that I was guided to follow.

"Sophia, I would often look at family and friends in long-term remission from addiction, and I would think, how did they do it? What made them successful at it? How many times did they have to start and stop their recovery before they knew it had to stick?

Gosh, I would be so jealous of them because I was never quite ready to commit to my recovery. And then, one day, I was. Is this how it works?" I asked.

Sophia replied, "Yes, that is exactly how it works. One day you hit rock bottom, and you have two choices: one is to return home to be with us in the non-physical world, and the other is to recover and live your mission. You chose your mission, and for that, we are grateful to you, Robin."

SEEKING ANSWERS

Stopping the generational trauma

Eighteen years ago, I took the brave step to meet with a food addiction specialist. It was the first time I was able to speak about my hidden shame. While I went to see her to work on my potential recovery, I know that I was there for an even more important reason. I asked her to show me how **not** to pass down this dreadful way of life to my children, to stop the trauma of addiction from my ancestry and in my family.

The food addiction specialist taught me how to speak with my children about food choices. She taught me how to help make my children self-responsible for having healthy lifestyles. This process worked. My children do gain weight like everyone else, but they also have the knowledge and drive to live healthy lifestyles. If they want to lose weight, they know how to do it in a healthy manner.

Is it safe to say that I have broken the generational obsessive-compulsive behavior in my family going forward? That is my prayer, for sure. In a healing session, I was told that this obsession goes back five generations. I know about my grandfather and grandmother, my mother, and myself, but I do not know the family history before that. Can you see a pattern in your family that might point to a generational behavior obsession? If so, when you heal your addictive nature, you are not only healing your family generations forward but also in generations back. How exciting would it be to become the hero of your family lineage?

My process of becoming the hero for my family lineage took years of peeling back the layers of wounds and maintaining a level of dysfunction that would be needed to bring me to this place of personal resolve eventually. What was the turning point that finally enabled me to go into recovery? The turning point was when I received a channeled message from my grandmother crying and apologizing for her part in my addiction. She also said that if I did not bury this addiction, my family would bury me. In the same reading, Sophia and Yeshua came in to say it was time to re-write this book in recovery.

Hitting rock bottom

Of course, the messages above should have been enough to stop my addictive behavior, right? No, I had to binge and purge one more time. This time there was blood coming out of both my nostrils. I had terrible pain in my lower back, my stomach, and my head. I knew that I had reached the end of my purging. I knew that if I continued to purge, I would die. Perhaps, this is what is referred to as "rock bottom."

According to Clearview Treatment Programs, "hitting rock bottom" is a phrase that almost everyone has heard when talking about the topic of addiction. For a phrase that is so important to the discussion of addiction, you may think that rock bottom could be easily defined or even simply identified. In actuality, rock bottom is a concept that means something different to every addict.

In the Clearview article, they share that:

> …rock bottom refers to a time or an event in life that causes an addict to reach the lowest possible point in their disease. It is a time when a person feels like things cannot get worse for them. Their life has been damaged so badly that it seems like there is nothing good left to destroy. Most addicts need to hit their own personal rock bottom before they can ever begin the addiction recovery process.

The key to understanding the concept of rock bottom is to be aware that it is a unique process for everyone. There are addicts who hit their rock bottom quickly. Others don't hit rock bottom for years. You don't need to focus on developing a bottom that looks like someone else's bottom. You don't need to sink to a specific deep, dark depth in your life to enter treatment. No matter what your rock bottom is, it's never too late to reach out and ask for help.

Creating a recovery plan

For me, the path to rock bottom was very slow. However, I can also say that I had been actively seeking help for 18 years. Beyond the Divine timing of living my Soul's journey to this point, is there a more human reason why attempts at recovery do not work? Getting clean from any addition takes great determination along with willpower, focus, perseverance, support, and—most importantly—a plan. Without a plan for recovery, the effort is destined to fail. A ship wouldn't set sail without a destination. A plane wouldn't leave the ground without a flight plan. So why do some recovering addicts feel as if they can negotiate their recovery from addiction without a plan? It's impossible.

A plan allows the recovering addict the best chance for success. A plan provides for the possibility of relapse but makes the recovering addict aware of the situations that may lead to a relapse. The article from Choices Recovery Center includes five critical reasons why recovery from addiction could fail:

1. *The Quick Fix.* Often addiction stems from looking for a "quick fix" to a problem, like taking an aspirin for a headache. But lasting recovery requires that we get out of this mindset and find other, more healthy ways to soothe ourselves and alleviate our pain.

2. *Unhealthy Behavior:* In recovery, we must make the changes to eliminate "triggers," and be hypersensitive about our environment and, at least initially, avoid contact with their

source of addiction. Not doing this can often be a sign that the recovery process is not working.

3. *Seeking Help:* The danger of isolation is greatest after treatment has ended for all recovering addicts. It is essential to keep the lines of communication open with a support group, counselor, family member, or therapist. Old addictive emotions and behaviors tend to build up until old habits surface.

4. *Hoping to Fail.* The process of recovery is ongoing and requires a lot of hard work and dedication. Many people in recovery want to be "*better*" already without having gone through all of the work it takes to get there. It is important to remember that a clean and sober person can be even more fun and more comfortable to be around.

5. *Recovery from Addiction.* One of the greatest dangers for a recovering addict, especially early in the recovery process, is to think, " I am healed." While it may not be required to take medicine or have to attend support groups for the rest of their lives, ongoing awareness of their mental and emotional state is what will maintain a clean and healthy quality of life.

The Choices Recovery article concludes by saying that "No recovery from addiction is without peril. Staying in tune with one's state of mind is the best way to gauge just where one is in the recovery process. A relapse can happen at any point. All recovery is ongoing, and no recovery is safe from relapse. By following a solid plan and maintaining due diligence, a recovering addict gives themselves the best chance for success."

Assembling my recovery team

While my first attempt at recovery was eighteen years ago, I have been following a steadier path for the past twelve years and a real dedication in the past three years. This path has included an integrative one of mind, body, spiritual, and emotional healing experiences. The journey began when I went to the Oneness University in India and started my "Inner Child" work. One does this type of emotional healing work to resolve the traumatic childhood emotions and experiences that your inner child still holds. The intention is to address the traumas and then to regain the joy, innocence, and confidence that were your birthright.

Mental and Emotional Healing

I talked a good talk about inner child work, went to many workshops, became certified in many modalities, and, yet, I was deeply in addiction. I finally declared that I was mentally and emotionally unstable, and I needed help. I then dived deeper into this work with my therapist over the past three years, expanding beyond my childhood into traumas from my teens, my young adult years, and now my mature adult years. Living an examined life is helping me to peel back the layers of my human psyche like a rose or an onion. At the core is your unique spirit or Soul. When you have peeled back enough layers, you can live in conscious awareness with your Soul. For mental and emotional work to hold for me, I had to ground my Soul in my body.

Energy Healing

As someone who spent her life abusing her body by purging, it would make sense that my Soul hung safely outside my body in my higher energy fields. Another vital part of my healing has been energy healing. Energy Healing is defined as a form of healing that manipulates, restores, or balances the flow of energy in the body. The energy is channeled through the practitioner to the client, helping remove energy deficiencies and blockages, which then activates the body's own natural ability to heal itself.

My energy healer was intrigued that I could do the work that I do as a spiritual messenger with my Soul living outside my body. She has worked diligently with me to ground my Soul but to also clear my energetic field of debris left by my life of humiliation and shame. With my Soul grounded in my body, life is so much more vibrant, and my work is so much more profound.

One of my most favorite forms of energy is the Japanese healing modality of Seimei, an invisible phenomenon that is of the non-physical world. Seimei is in all people and things, so it is in this world but not of it. It is considered a spiritual, result-oriented science based on a tangible outcome. Seimei is a holistic solution for issues ranging from acute pain (such as post-operative), sports injuries, or the flu to more chronic symptoms such as accident trauma, migraines, neck and back discomfort/pain, and everything in between. Seimei sessions have removed imbalances in my energetic field and my physical body.

Physical Healing

As previously described in the book, my naturopath intuited that I may not be producing dopamine in my brain and tested me for this. The test resulted in a diagnosis that lead me to a natural remedy to increase the dopamine in my brain that I do not produce naturally. Dopamine is required to find feelings of joy within yourself and not look for pleasure in outside substances. Is low dopamine is a trigger for addiction? My naturopath works with me to ensure that my body is receiving all of the natural supplements and vitamins it needs to maintain a healthy environment. When I feel healthy and happy, I am not reaching for sugar.

Another vital part of my physical healing is massage. In a massage, I follow my massage therapist's every movement, and I send light to those parts of my body for healing. I share sincere gratitude for my body for carrying my Soul in this lifetime. As you can see, this is a full reversal for someone who abused her body. In gratitude for my body, I find the grace inherent in my body. In recovery, having a massage can be the trigger for the release of "feel-good" hormones.

According to the American Massage Therapy Association, massage helps to increase serotonin and dopamine (feel-good hormones) and decrease cortisol, which is related to stress. During detox and withdrawal, dopamine levels drop dramatically, making for uncomfortable or even painful sensations. Therapeutic massage focuses on the body's pressure points, which are linked to the brain's vagus nerve. Massage can also help lower heart rate and blood pressure.

The last member of my formal healing team is my general allopathic practitioner. This role is to check whether there was any physical damage to my organs after years of purging. After extensive bloodwork and heart testing, there were no signs of lasting impact on my physical body.

Other members of my healing team include all my family and friends to whom I have entrusted my story. Their love and support let me know that I matter and that my presence in their life is essential. This feeling of belonging stops me from experiencing a deep sense of loneliness that can overcome me at times.

For fifteen years, my dog, Hailey, had been with me on every stage of this healing journey and was my angel at my feet. During the summer of finishing this book, Hailey left her physical vessel. It was a profound and deeply felt loss by our entire family. I was so distraught that Yeshua returned to say, "Put the *Feast & Famine* manuscript down for now. Mourn your loss fully. When the time is right to begin again, you will know."

Assemble your support team.

I would invite you to assemble a support team for your life. Yes, my team is robust, and I am deeply grateful that I have found each one of them. It takes a village to raise one's vibration, heal your physical and emotional wounds, live happily in the present moment in recovery, and plan for a future in remission. However, if you do not have the financial resources or access to an outstanding human healing team, there is always your Divine team on call in Spirit waiting to help. What I know for sure is that we are never alone and that through our Divine team, we can live a life of deep spiritual connection.

In my life, this deep connection has been both enjoyable and frustrating at the same time. The frustrating part came because I could not believe that any Divine Master would want to hang out with me, the addict. And yet, even at the height of my addiction, they presented me with wisdom, miracles, and unconditional love. This incredible energy that emanates from my Divine nature in connection with my Divine Source is beyond description. If I had to choose comparable earthly moments, I would say it was how I felt the first time I held my children or how I felt when I looked into Ori's eyes during our marriage ceremony. I can also find these moments in a spectacular sunrise or sunset

The Divine speaks to us in so many ways. If you want to learn how to connect to your Divine team, then I would recommend my second book, *The Divine Keys*. This simple book shares eighteen ways to live a Divinely guided life. This path has been a gift to me in many ways, and the most significant one is my ability to communicate with the Divine Masters. Sometimes I forget how extraordinary this is. Recently, I was reminded by my daughter, Gaby, of how strangers just come up to talk to me. This happens because I carry the light of the Divine, and so when I glance at them or smile at them, they know that their Divinity is being reflected back to them.

Although I now had many more answers about my addiction, I realized I'd need to take a deeper dive into my subconscious to prepare for writing this book fully. The next chapter deals with how I looked deeper into a past-life.

"Sophia, what can you share that would enable others to believe that our Soul has lived many lifetimes and that our Soul has a desire to learn specific outcomes in each one?" I asked.

"Yes, Robin, this is an easy topic for some and a very difficult topic for others. The purpose of each incarnation is to grow further your knowing that you are the Divine in a human body. There is no one better or worse than you. Each one of you is here experiencing what is required for you to learn on your journey.

And yes, the topic of the next chapter is one that triggers great anger and shame on this planet. A global reaction was precisely what was needed for humanity to grow as a species at the time."

HEALING PAST AND PRESENT LIFETIMES

Revealing your Soul's records

The Akashic Records contain the past, present, and future lifetime information of our Souls. Our Akashic Records are accessed by individuals who have been called to read the records. These records are like the Internet of the spiritual realm. If you desire information about your past lives, this lifetime, and perhaps a future lifetime, the Akashic Records contain this information. The majority of my private client work is done within the Akashic Records. Therefore, I was excited to bring my Akashic Records teacher to my community to teach her program. The information I received for my own life was extraordinary that weekend.

Past life memories

As I sat across from a student in the Akashic Records certification class, the student opened my Akashic Records, and she went back to one of my past lives. She said, "You were in the Holocaust." I was stunned to know that my most recent past life was so recent. She continued to say, "I see you at Auschwitz, with your two children, a girl, and a boy. You are all starving because of the minuscule amount of food that you receive. When you are given your food, your children hastily eat their share, and you eat your portion reluctantly because you would rather share your food with your children, but the guards are watching everyone eat.

So, you hastily eat yours as well. As soon as the guards left, you would throw up your food and feed it to your children."

When the student told me this, I felt like a mother bird giving worms to her babies. I wasn't ready to allow myself to relive this past life energetically. The feeling of knowing that I would have to experience my children again starving to death would have been excruciating. To feel my experience of the Holocaust would have been crushing—and, to be honest, I was not ready to do that. I just took her word for it, as she seemed sincere. I then shared with the student my lifelong affliction with bulimia. Sharing my addiction was a big step for me since I had never told anyone other than my family or friends.

She welcomed my sharing with a compassionate look, and she said, "In your Holocaust lifetime, what you did by vomiting your food was a gift to your children. You may heal your addiction to vomiting in this lifetime if you choose to do so." In retrospect, it seemed so logical that I vomited to save my children in a terrible situation. I am blessed not to be persecuted in this lifetime, and yet I created a life of humiliation and shame just to keep on vomiting. This student reader's insights suggested to me that traumas from our past lives can impact our current lifetime.

In my work in the Akashic Records, I have seen this play out many times. A chronic backache in this lifetime could be a knife wound from a past life. Holding onto excess weight in this lifetime could be due to a past life of starvation. These two examples presume that we have lived other lifetimes and that we return to heal past traumas in this lifetime. Before our reincarnation, our Soul determines what it wants to learn in this lifetime and then calls in other Souls to play significant roles in our current lives.

As your Soul guides your life, you have an opportunity to release past-life traumas that are held in your subconscious mind. After that class, I wondered when I would be ready to release my trauma from the Holocaust. I continued to suffer deeply with bulimia, and then, suddenly, one day, I found myself ready to do the inner work that would lead me to a resolution. I asked a dear spiritual friend to make a referral for me to do the healing required to live a life with a healthy relationship with food. She referred me to her therapist mentor, and I set up an appointment.

Taking the next steps

When I arrived at the appointment, I was stunned to see that my new therapist mentor was none other than the student reader from the Akashic Records class! If you did not believe in Divine synchronicity up to this point, I invite you to do so now. How could this not have been arranged by the spiritual realm? Even my skeptics would have to agree. And so, my journey with Kathleen Humpage began.

Kathleen and I spent a year dancing around the subject until I was ready to dive deeper into my Holocaust past life. When the Nazis captured my family, my husband was sent to the gas chambers first. My children and I lasted longer in this evil place until my children were taken from me and brought to the gas chambers. From that moment on, I was filled with the most extraordinary grief imaginable. I continued to throw up my rations until the day I turned towards the wall while lying down in my barrack shelf, and I died from grief and starvation.

I grieved the loss of my family deeply in my therapist mentor's office that day, feeling every horrible pain of deprivation and unimaginable loss. I thought I was done with bulimia, and yet there was much more to learn. I was still not complete. The healing of any significant trauma comes in layers. To this day, I am still haunted by the vision of the barracks and the inhumanity to man, woman, and child that I witnessed every day.

Many other authors have so eloquently explained the horror of that experience. One of my favorite books on the topics was written from an author's past-life regression sessions. The book is called *The Angel of Auschwitz: A Spiritual Memoir of Forgiveness and Healing*. This book tells the story of the spiritual healers who were present in the Holocaust. I feel a kinship with the author, Tarra Light. She also was in the Holocaust and came back to share her story of healing, compassion, and forgiveness. I envied her ability to write her book from this place, and it would take years of healing work before I could experience any of those three attributes.

One year later, I was sitting across from Kathleen in her office, and I said, "It is time to go back to the Holocaust." I closed my eyes and returned to the tortures of the Holocaust. I felt the pain of the loss of the six million Jews and others who perished in the Holocaust. As I stayed present with the pain, my mentor shared that she could see millions of Souls standing around me. She said that each one had a name written across their Being. I said, "Those are the six million who suffered as I did in Nazi Germany." When thinking about Souls sharing their names, it seemed important at the time to recognize them as individuals, not as just the collective six million. Each one of them had a unique Soul and a distinct life experience. By lumping them together, we certainly create numerical impact, but on this particular day, they wanted me to know that they were individuals, too.

Where do I go from here?

On this day in Kathleen's office, I acknowledged my pain, allowed the suffering from my past life to heal, and began the healing of bulimia in my current life. I declared that I would do my part to heal the lives of my husband and my children and our ancestors. I declared that I would do my part to heal the collective lineage of those who suffered in the Holocaust and those who continue to remember the atrocities that occurred. We shall never forget, but we can heal. With this acknowledgment, the assembled six million Souls faded back into All Being, and I began my journey to heal my daily struggle with bulimia and to activate my relationship with Sophia.

I knew that I had to come into recovery from addiction and that I still had lingering anger about the Holocaust. In spiritual healing, you must come into forgiveness to truly heal from trauma. It is important to note that forgiveness does not mean that you condone another person's behavior. How was I supposed to forgive and have compassion for the Nazis who killed my family? In a healing session with a different colleague, she said, "Don't you think they were just doing the best that they could?"

I replied, "Hell, no, I don't! I think they were soulless, heartless bastards."

She replied, "Can you say that they were following orders?" I capitulated on that excuse; if I could accept that they were just following orders, then maybe I could come into forgiveness, even though I could never find compassion for them. Where was their compassion? I presume I will never know the answer to that question, but from having expressed forgiveness, I now could finish writing *Feast & Famine*.

It is my privilege to share with you more about the Mother of Creation, Sophia, and her assistance in my healing in the upcoming chapters.

Sophia's Insights for Chapter Eleven

"Finally, it is your turn," I said to Sophia.

*"Ha, it has been my turn way before this page in the book,"
she replied. "I have been with you, Robin, since the very
beginning of your addiction, and I have been with you
throughout your journey of pain to suffering to surrender
to grace. We are grateful that you have taken this journey
with us and that you have the courage to bare your Soul
in the book."*

*After some thought, I concluded that there is no more
hiding for me after writing this book. When I shared the
idea of "no more hiding" with a dear spiritual sister, she
replied, "This is no longer the time or place for hiding. The
world needs all of us to stand in our truth."*

CHAPTER ELEVEN

SOPHIA AND THE DIVINE FEMININE

The Divine Feminine

If you have studied the Old or the New Testaments, you've learned that humanity was created in the image of God. What is the image of God or the image of the Divine? In my view, it is the perfect alignment of Divine Feminine and Divine Masculine energies. What would happen if humanity was able to live fully in both its Divine Feminine and Masculine traits and become enlightened? The answer is that through this new-found sense of personal and global unity, we would no longer need the divisive system called "religion."

Thousands of years ago, to maintain control of the masses, religious leaders attempted to diminish the Divine Feminism (Sophia) within the pages of scripture. Or did they? In Judaism, the Divine Feminine is called the *Shechinah,* the feminine manifestation, aspect, or *emanation* of God, as the Kabbalists say. In other words, God's presence in our world, giving life to all beings, is referred to as She or the *Shechinah.* When referring to God's transcendence beyond this world, God is written as He. God's presence on this earth is described in Judaism through the Divine Feminine, and his presence beyond our human knowing is described through the Divine Masculine.

In Christianity, She is called the Holy Spirit, a nondescript, ghost-like Being. I find it interesting that no one I have asked knows what or who the Holy Spirit is. Sophia is the Holy Spirit. She has been hiding in plain sight, given top billing, and no one knows who she is. "The Father, the Son, and the Holy Spirit" is the most common way to refer to the holy trinity in Christianity. The Holy Trinity is described as the *mystery of three* in one God: the Father, the Son, and the Holy Spirit. For example, Christians are directed to baptize in the name of the Father, Son, and Holy Spirit. The phrase clearly says *in the name of,* not in *their* names, because this is only one God expressed in three ways. We have been clearly shown who the Father and the Son are, but who is the Holy Spirit?

Defining the energy of Creation

She is Sophia, and she is best known as Holy Grace, Holy Wisdom, the Divine Mother, and the Divine Feminine. She has also referred to herself as the Creatrix of All Being. Therefore, the energy of Sophia is Creation. When we welcome Sophia into our lives, we are opening to a life of more magnificent creation, of freedom, of independence. It would make sense that, if biblical leaders felt that humanity needed to be controlled at that time, it would be best to place the energy of Sophia in the veiled sections of the biblical texts.

In Joyce Rupp's article, "Desperately Seeking Sophia," I learned a great deal about the biblical background of Sophia. Rupp writes that the biblical Sophia is more than a metaphor; she is an expression of the presence of God. She discusses how Sophia is most often described as Holy Wisdom in the Bible. Rupp writes, "Some passages speak of wisdom as a quality or a truth to guide our lives. Here wisdom is presented as a 'thing'— such as wise sayings, proverbs, and moral exhortations. There are many other passages, however, that refer to wisdom as a person. It is here that the feminine pronoun is always used and is consistently reflective of the Divine presence. This wisdom is Holy Wisdom: Hagia Sophia."

Rupp supports my conclusion that Sophia was ultimately hidden from us to ensure that the masculine influence was more potent in the Christian religion and to remove any connection to other feminine-based philosophies or religious practices. Most importantly, Rupp and I agree that Sophia's energy is so powerful that any attempts to separate us from our genuine connection will fail. Rupp summarizes her article by reminding us that Sophia will not fail us. She will always draw us deeper and further, for there is no end to the mystery of her life with us.

Welcoming Sophia into my life

When did Sophia begin to draw me deeper into a connection with her and the Divine Feminine wisdom? My in-depth learning process started after the incredible spiritual event on the planet when we reached the end of the Mayan calendar on December 21, 2012, and entered what has been called The Golden Age or The Age of Aquarius. The message I consistently heard in the materials I studied at that time was that we had entered a new age of God. We were leaving the Age of Man (one that lacked balance between male and female and one that was based on power and profits, without regard for Mother Earth and all of her inhabitants.) It was time to raise the vibration of the feminine on the planet.

Many of my spiritual colleagues were chanting, "Up with the Feminine and Down with the Masculine." I knew that the feminine rising <u>above</u> the masculine was not what was required now. As a participant in the Women's Liberation Movement, I knew that the most significant growth for all of humanity (especially women) would come in the form of honoring of feminine and masculine, our unity of male and female, our Oneness with all Divine Beings.

In my heart, I knew that for us to reach this place of Oneness with ourselves and within our world, we must first awaken the Divine Feminine on our planet. I believe that my intensive study of this topic is what enabled Sophia to connect with me to write this book. If you are interested in studying this topic more deeply, I would recommend *The Sophia Code* by Kaia Ra and *Return of the Divine Sophia* by Tricia McCannon.

The impact of Archetypal patterns

Another area of study that has been important to me is the archetype definitions shared by Carl Jung. He developed archetypes as a way of thinking about the psychological and emotional qualities of thought and behavior that is common across all of humanity. A Divine Feminine archetype exhibits the best and highest expression of these energies in both women and men.

In this new age of God called The Golden Age, we are required to place an equal emphasis on the feminine energies to balance the masculine energies ruling the world at this time. To be clear, both men and women carry within their psyche, both Divine Masculine and Divine Feminine archetypal energies. In addition, archetypes have both light (positive) and shadow (negative) influences on our lives.

For this book, we will focus on the following feminine archetypes paraphrased from a post from www.innergoddess.com:

Goddess/Creatrix Archetype: Highly spiritual creator and manifestor. Possesses high intuitive wisdom and radiates unconditional love. (Shadow attribute: Do I doubt myself or the Divine?)

Queen/Leader Archetype: Selfless and wise. Accepts reality and lives in the present moment. Lives life fully and desires Unity in her world. (Shadow attribute: Do I choose suffering over leading myself or others?)

Lover Archetype: Passionate about life. Sensitive, compassionate, and kind. Loves contact and connection. (Shadow attribute: Do I compare myself to others and focus on our differences?)

Mother Archetype: Provides loving care and well-being for her family. Nurturing and stabilizing influence. (Shadow attribute: Do I nurture others over nurturing myself?)

Priestess Archetype: Intuitive awareness of other dimensions and realms. Connected to her body and searches for higher wisdom. (Shadow attribute: Do I trust the answers that I receive from the Divine?)

Warrioress Archetype: Stands and fights for the truth. Assertive, courageous, and protects the innocent. (Shadow attribute: Do I create chaos and withhold love from myself and others?)

I trust that you can see these archetypes reflected in your own life, whether you are a male or female. Quite often, the shadow aspect is reflected by those closest to us. This quote from Carl Yung says it quite clearly, "Everything that irritates us about others can lead us to an understanding of ourselves."

Welcome Sophia into your life.

Now that you are more knowledgeable about Sophia's Divine Feminine nature, I invite you to recognize her presence in your own life. In essence, I invite you to identify the beauty in your life. Notice the snowflakes in the air or pray for others. These simple acts are the presence of grace in your life. See the world through the eyes of Sophia, speak to others as Sophia, and take the right actions to bring blessing to yourself and others.

"Happy is the person who meditates on Sophia, who reflects in one's heart on Sophia's ways and ponders her secrets, pursuing her like a hunter, and lying in wait on her paths." (Sirach 15:20–22).

The following chapters in the book will define a healing path that Sophia shared with me to support my journey to recovery from bulimia. You may have heard these steps in other programs. Who is not to say that Sophia did not guide these blessed Souls to know these healing truths?

Sophia's Insights for Chapter Twelve

"Sophia, what can you share with us about pain that could prevent us from turning pain into suffering?" I asked.

Sophia replied, "You have an interesting phrase on the earth plane: there are only two events you can count on happening, and they are death and taxes."

Clearly, you can count on pain, too. I am not saying that to make you feel worse. I am saying that to relax you into the pain because it is inevitable.

Do what you can to heal it and do not allow it to consume you. It is in pain's consumption of you that suffering begins. Most important, you cannot recover from a place of focusing on the pain.

You must focus on the healing and how you will feel when the pain is gone. This simple manifesting tool can help you to not move into suffering even if you are in great pain."

CHAPTER TWELVE

PAIN IS INEVITABLE

Pay attention to pain

Being a human being is complicated. Each one of us is comprised of four parts: mind, body, spirit, and emotion. Any event that impacts one of the components has an indirect effect on all the other components. For example, if you are injured physically, then you will have mental anguish or perhaps emotional turmoil. The question that we must explore is this: how does pain serve your life? In an article in *Psychology Today*, Dr. Ana Nogales writes that "Pain is our body's way of informing us that something is wrong. We must pay attention to it. The way we live, combined with what we eat, affects our central nervous system, which affects our perception of pain."

In her article, Dr. Nogales addresses the impact of addiction on pain. She shares that "if we add other factors, such as smoking, drinking, or the consumption of other drugs, we have to ask ourselves why we willingly harm ourselves. However, there are other ways to get the same benefits without exposing oneself to the harmful effects of drug or alcohol use." Dr. Nogales makes relevant recommendations like staying active through exercise and building up our endurance through increasing our efforts over time. In the article, she writes about how people are afraid of getting hurt and dealing with more pain through exercise. For many, the opposite is true; being inactive typically leads to more pain over time. She reminds us that when we are not sleeping well, our bodies undergo stress, and a person becomes more irritable.

Understanding how pain impacts our lives

Dr. Nogales expresses how pain significantly impacts our lives. With the limited activity that occurs as a result of pain, a person will likely become pessimistic about one's future. Anxiety and depression are common responses to pain, which, unfortunately, intensify our suffering. She reminds us that our thoughts affect the way we feel. Negative thoughts can be a form of physical and emotional torture. The Universe will provide us with whatever we are focused on. Therefore, if you are focusing on pain, you will receive more ways to be in pain. Pain is a beautiful sign that you need help. Seek the advice that you need.

And lastly, she asks us to understand our pain. "Learn to deal with it through relaxation exercises, deep breathing, meditation, prayer – whatever it is that brings you peace. However, don't believe everything you think, as our thoughts are sometimes deceiving. Mindfully review your thoughts, and you will see how reality can distort what you think, which generates unnecessary stress, which in and of itself creates further tension and affects our perception of our pain."

Reduce the opportunity for pain by getting adequate rest

For me, pain has served in two very clear ways. I have this expression, "Spirit took me out." This action by Spirit is in direct response to whenever I have been moving too fast in my life, and I need to slow down. The way the Divine slows me down is by making me stay in bed for a few days. This slow down could manifest in the form of an illness or injury. Why do I let it get this far, that I would need to be "taken out"? That is simple: I am not paying sufficient attention to my integrated systems and, therefore, I do not see that I need to rest.

Early on in my career as an Akashic Record reader, a woman came to me for a session. As I opened her records, I heard nothing. Almost panicking, I began to do some energy healing on her as an alternative to reading her Akashic Records. As I moved around her, I saw four letters appear on her chest: R E S T. I sat back down in my chair, and I said, "I am sorry, I am only receiving one word from the records: "Rest."

She opened her eyes and looked at me and said, "I told you that I came here to understand what is next in my life now that I am retired for six months, but what I did not tell you is that my husband and I divorced, and my daughter has been very ill in the past six months, too. What I came here for is permission to rest."

The benefits of adequate rest

The idea of resting is challenging for us in our crazy, hectic lives, but it's probably one of the essential parts of our lives if we want to be effective in serving others. Adequate rest enables us to perform at our optimal best. Can you imagine a day without coffee, tea, or chocolate to keep you going? Indeed, many recognize that meditation, exercise, and healthy eating are all key components for limiting the pain that is inevitable in our lives. So what are the reasons that we don't value our rest? According to *Psychology Today*, most of us believe that if we rest, we are unproductive and lazy. In fact, many people think of resting as death! Have you ever heard that expression, "I will rest when I am dead"? Ironically, death may happen sooner than later with that attitude!

Rest is the springboard for daily alignment

Resting enables our entire system to rejuvenate and begin each day in a state of alignment. When you first wake up, it is a wonderful time to meditate or pray for all the abundance that you can envision coming your way on that day. According to the teachings of the global Law of Attraction teachers, Abraham-Hicks, 17 seconds of pure thought is the "ignition point" of manifesting, which means if you hold a thought for 17 seconds, you set in motion its manifestation. The purpose behind this rule of thumb is to get you to think purely for 17 seconds and to have that desire become stronger as you work up to holding that thought-desire for a full 68 seconds. Each fourth of that 68 seconds gets more potent than the last, thereby creating a compelling point of attraction.

What happens when we don't rest?

When we are "unrested," we do stupid things. We trip and fall because our mind is moving faster than our bodies. We make impulsive decisions that we regret. We eat crappy, low-energy food, thinking that we will get a rush of adrenaline to move forward in our day. And if you are reading this book because you are bulimic, well, you know what we do when our bodies are filled with crappy food… purge, right?

Over time, a lack of rest, insufficient exercise, unhealthy food, and overuse of supplements to compensate for these other inadequacies will wreak havoc on all of your integrated systems. It would be like never putting oil in your car engine, then putting in the cheapest gas you can, and never changing the tires. Would you expect your car to run at optimal capacity for you? Then, why do that to your own vessel and its integrated systems?

Lack of rest leads to burnout

In an article from Paracelsus Recovery, the author looks at burnout as an underlying cause of addiction. The article describes burnout as severe exhaustion that comes from our highly stressful and demanding lives. "Over time, this relentless drive can take its toll. People with severe burnout feel overwhelmed with stress when they wake up in the morning and when they climb into bed at night. Burnout can be intense enough to threaten health, relationships, and careers. Sometimes, it drags on for years while people continue to push through feelings of severe mental, physical, and emotional exhaustion. Burnout can be measured using specialized lab tests such as Cortisol levels. Cortisol is produced by the adrenal glands to protect the body against stress, and it gets fatigued and literally 'burnt out' when stress is ongoing."

Burnout leads to secondary addiction

Burnout can lead to disruptions in sleep patterns. One might think that burnout would make it easier to sleep because a person who is in burnout is so darn tired. The opposite usually occurs; racing thoughts prevent the person from going to sleep and then wake up in the middle of the night. How would a person alleviate sleeplessness? Perhaps turn to a sleeping pill or alcohol. This cycle of lack of sleep relieved by an addictive substance is a path that can lead to an unproductive life. People wake up from the sedatives or alcohol with drowsiness and a foggy mind. Some people rely on caffeine, food, cocaine, or amphetamines to be productive in their day. Because none of the addictive distractions above actually solves burnout, it is possible to see how by choosing a distraction, one can spiral into a full-fledged substance addiction.

Other signs and symptoms of burnout

The Paracelsus Recovery article shares signs and symptoms to watch for if concerned that you may be suffering from burnout:

- Weakened immunity and frequent minor illnesses such as colds, headaches, allergies or skin irritations
- Difficulty with decision-making (even in people who are usually very decisive)
- Feelings of physical, mental and emotional exhaustion
- Loss of interest in normally enjoyable activities, including sexuality
- Feelings of dissatisfaction, disillusionment, and boredom, or a sense that life has lost meaning and purpose
- Intense emotions, including depressive thoughts, anxiety, and panic
- Loss of self-confidence and self-esteem
- Anger and irritability, frequent bursts of anger

Seeking help and support is essential

If you are experiencing the signs of burnout, get help to seek out solutions for your exhaustion, manage your workload, require more of your partner, friends, and family. Ideally, you would seek out the support of a skilled therapist to learn techniques to manage your stress and create new ways to feel joy and success in your life. If your burnout is complicated by drug or alcohol abuse, seek the help you need at support groups or rehab center. It is essential to restore your depleted cells and boost your adrenal function. Holistic medical professionals are ideally suited for this type of protocol.

Even if we follow all the rules of health and wellness, pain is inevitable. Beyond our complicated mind, body, spirit, and emotional system, other people in our lives impact us negatively in our personal and professional lives. Therefore, on planet earth, pain is unavoidable and inevitable.

Though pain is an unavoidable part of life on this planet, the good news is that suffering is optional. Just when you thought there might not be much more to say about suffering, I have dedicated a chapter to it!

"Sophia, when I share this next answer from you with others, everyone—and I mean everyone—looks like they just received the most important aha! truth in their life," I shared.

Sophia smiled and said, "Indeed, this is very powerful and life-altering.

There is only one primary addiction on your planet, and that addiction is to suffering. Once you are caught in the trap of suffering, you will have to choose a secondary addiction to keep on suffering.

This secondary addiction can be a substance, a relationship, a belief pattern, or a lifestyle. There is no shortage of 'tools' to stay in suffering on your planet.

When you are ready to love yourself, you will choose a healthier path for your life that does not include suffering."

SUFFERING IS AN OPTION

Pain and suffering are two different events.

The first time I heard the expression, "suffering is an option," I was at the Oneness University in India doing deep inner child work. I was reliving all of the known sufferings in my life. It made me wonder how suffering could be an option if we are all exposed to so much of it? Perhaps, we place so much emphasis on suffering because we lump pain and suffering into the same sentence. "Oh, that poor soul, she has so much pain and suffering." "He must be suffering, so; he is in excruciating pain." Pain is inevitable; that has been established! But is suffering the necessary outcome of pain? Many spiritual teachers would say one has nothing to do with the other. When we learn to separate and distinguish between the two, we will be so much happier.

In her *New York Times* best-selling book *Why People Don't Heal and How They Can*, Carolyn Myss writes:

> We are not meant to stay wounded. We are supposed to move through our tragedies and challenges and to help each other move through the many painful episodes of our lives. By remaining stuck in the power of our wounds, we block our own transformation. We overlook the greater gifts inherent in our wounds—the strength to overcome them and the lessons that we are meant to receive through them. Wounds are the means through which we enter the hearts of other people. They are meant to teach us to become compassionate and wise.

Being in pain may not lead to suffering.

Can you imagine someone in pain still being able to be a happy person? Is it possible that they have figured out that pain is heightened by layering suffering on top of it? Perhaps they have chosen not to be miserable and have their mindset on their wellness. If you believe in the Law of Attraction, you will call in and receive more misery if you are miserable. We get what we focus our attention on. Why, then, do we choose to suffer? At the core of every outward addiction is an underlying addiction to suffering. Even if you get your outward addiction under control, you need to heal the underlying addiction to suffering.

Addicted to suffering

Your addiction to suffering can come in many forms. For example, in my life, I struggled with the pain of disappointment. I know that disappointment is a form of suffering because the Divine asked me to let go of it. One night, while I was lying in bed, the Divine shared, "Release the Disappointment." I began releasing the emotional charge around all the ways that other people had disappointed me. After I was complete, the Divine said, "That was a good start. How about releasing the disappointment in yourself?"

Let me count the ways! As a person who has specialized in being my own victim and persecutor, I had much disappointment in myself. This addictive behavior that I had mastered perpetuated so much disappointment in myself. I knew that I must eat healthily to fulfill my Divine mission, and yet, at the drop of a hat, I could find myself not eating healthy. Here is an example of the voice in my head that would immediately start a dialogue with me in my addictive state:

Inner Addict: "What do you want to eat?"

Me: "Something healthy."

Inner Addict: "Yes, but wouldn't you rather have this unhealthy food?"

Me: "Of course, I would, but I have to maintain my energy, my vessel, and my emotional peace of mind."

Inner Addict: "Come on, you can eat this crappy food, and then you can throw up."

Me: "Okay, let's eat a small amount of crappy food."

Inner Addict: "Okay, we can eat a little bit of it, and then the rest can be healthy."

Me: "Damn, I just ate the whole thing, and now I can give myself permission to eat a ton more until I am so sick of myself, I will throw up."

Inner Addict: "Gotcha."

Me: "You suck, Robin, I am so disappointed in you."

Letting go of suffering

What did it take for me to give up my suffering in the form of disappointment? The simple answer was to eat healthily, exercise, rest, and drink water. Being healthy was just as much of an option in my life as was suffering. The battle was with my inner addict, who would undermine me every time. Why was that? Because by empowering my inner addict, I chose to stay hidden and to live in fear.

The inner addict was like a dark knight encased in shining armor. The dark knight declared, "I will protect you from even greater forms of disappointment and hurts in the world. I will ensure that you cannot move past your disappointment and that you don't have to take any risks and that you can live a small, insignificant life. If you move beyond your inner addict, then how can I protect you from being hurt and disappointed?"

The highly regarded spiritual teacher, Thich Nhat Hanh, says that "People have a hard time letting go of their suffering. Out of a fear of the unknown, they prefer suffering that is familiar." I would take that one step further and say that suffering is a habit. We wake up in the morning, and we have a choice to set our day to be one without suffering or one with suffering.

The recognition of which day it will be is simple: if you wake up obsessing about what's wrong, you will suffer. If you wake up thinking about how blessed you are, you have a much higher chance of not suffering that day. Suffering becomes either an unconscious habit or, once we're aware of the habit, it becomes a conscious choice to avoid.

Choosing not to suffer

In choosing not to suffer, you must also choose to own your pain. Choosing begins with the acknowledgment that you genuinely have a problem that needs to be dealt with. This deep understanding of the cause of your suffering empowers you or fortifies you with the courage to move into the next phase of surrender.

In my own life, I had to acknowledge that I didn't truly love myself or my relationship with my Divine more than my relationship with the significant people in my life. I was expecting them to love me enough to feel better about myself. The level of pain that I was carrying could never be healed by anyone but myself in relationship with myself and with my Divine.

By relying on others, I set myself up for other forms of deep disappointment, which, in turn, created great sadness within me. What does a sad person often like to do? Listen to their inner addict, of course. I was so sad that I thought that milk chocolate would make me feel better. In reality, the caffeine and the sugar in milk chocolate made me feel physically worse and emotionally defeated.

I am not saying that I had to give up chocolate. I had to find other options like a darker chocolate or cacao raw desserts. For sure, milk chocolate is a bulimia trigger for me. Even today, milk chocolate is like a drug to me. In my active addiction, I could guarantee that if I had milk chocolate, I would have a 100 percent chance of bingeing and then a 100 percent chance of purging. Today, in recovery, I may still have the same statistic for bingeing, but 0 percent for purging.

Knowing that is the case, why would I still eat it? Because I know I will gravitate to it in moments of emotional weakness. Just like any other addict, I should have a choice to give in or not. So was I addicted to the chocolate or the suffering? Perhaps both. The chocolate itself has addictive ingredients, and it did make me feel good temporarily. But my real addiction was to suffering through the ensuing disappointment with myself.

What does suffering teach us?

Could there be a benefit to suffering in our lives? My teachers from India, SriAmmaBhagavan, had asked all their students to become, "Agents of Suffering." To be honest, when I first heard this, I thought that was a ridiculous request—why would they want us to suffer? Having suffered so profoundly, I can now say that suffering is an amazing teacher.

If you are open to exploring your suffering by truly feeling the pain, a world of understanding of the root causes of your suffering will become available to you. From this understanding of the root cause of your suffering, you will be ready to surrender your suffering. The next step on Sophia's Divine Path to Healing, *Surrender is Required* is not just a declaration of the words, "I surrender my suffering." You have to mean it with your entire heart. The Divine will know whether you truly mean it or if you are just tired of suffering.

Why would anyone hold onto suffering? The answer is simple: because you believe you still need it. You may be holding onto the negative attention-getting behavior to get *some* kind of attention, or perhaps you are not ready to receive positive attention in your life. When you truly surrender to the Divine, you have to be ready to ultimately live a life of fulfilling your own needs and desires. If not, you will need to go back and dig deeper into your pain to understand how it continues to serve you. What are you afraid of? How do you need to protect yourself? These questions are not intended to shame you but to help you to know yourself. You will know when the time is right for true surrender. As Buddha shared, "*Suffering is not holding you; you are holding suffering.*"

Suffering is an option – meaning you can always suffer if you want to. However, if you don't want to suffer, then surrender is required. I share more about surrender in the next chapter.

"Sophia, coming to this chapter in my second re-write of this book, I was riveted by the anger I heard in my voice about surrender in the first draft of the book.

I was stuck on whether I should delete this chapter and start again. What I decided is that I would keep my initial chapter and then write more from my current perspective. I could see how much I had shifted on my journey."

Sophia replied, "Yes, Robin, life is a constant unraveling of what was, while at the exact time, an unfolding of what is to come. This unraveling and unfolding require that you live in the present moment to experience all of the movement with us.

As we have shared before, connection to the spiritual realm and the resulting grace can only occur in present-moment awareness. Surrender your pain, my dear ones, grace is here."

SURRENDER IS REQUIRED

This chapter is written from two different points in time. The first part was from when I was in active addiction, and the second is from a place of recovery. I hope that you can see the difference between surrender in addiction and surrender in recovery to your own life.

Surrender from Addiction

I was leaving to drive to Maine to pick up our son, Garrett, for spring break. My relationship with my husband, Ori, felt like there was a distance between us. I decided to tell him how I felt. He had just finished an extensive list of household chores, and this was not the right time to talk with him about our relationship. We both lost our temper, and he stormed out of the kitchen to take a shower.

He yelled from the shower, "Here you go again, looking for a reason to get all worked up so that you can obsess about us and ruin your trip to Maine."

I screamed an obsenity at him and stormed out of the house without saying goodbye. That was a big deal to me because I am always saying "I love you" and "goodbye" in case it is the very last time I should see him. I jumped in the car and started driving.

When I was packing earlier in the morning, I was looking around my office for a book on tape to listen to in the car. I reached for the CD series, *Women, Food and God* by Geneen Roth. I picked it up and put it in my PC bag. Determined to have a productive, peaceful, and joyful time away, I began to listen to the CD series. Little did I know that the fight with Ori and listening to this CD series was a set-up from Spirit.

Talking directly to me

From the very first word, I knew that Geneen Roth was talking to me. I discovered that I was an obsessive-compulsive overeater. The more spiritual I became, the more my obsessive behavior was triggered. My work requires me to be comfortable with myself and my body. And when I am not comfortable, I bolt—just like I did from our home. Becoming comfortable with my body—the one that I had abused my entire adult life—seemed like an impossible task.

What I know for sure about my Divine journey is that I must keep my Soul energy in my vessel. You know, the one with the fat belly. And speaking of my stomach, I must meditate by focusing my attention on my fat, disgusting belly. You know, the one that I don't even want my husband or a medical professional to touch. That one. The one that holds my Soul.

Yes, I must be in a relationship with my belly every day during meditation because I must focus my energy inside myself to bring Heaven to Earth. Then I thought: "What a joke, heaven to earth. Why would Divine energy want to live in this body? This fat, old, out-of-shape, abused, unloved, and unwanted body."

Ready, set, bolt

I discovered in Roth's book that gals like me—deep on their spiritual path—will bolt as fast as a shot away from themselves as soon as they become vulnerable. Yup, I opened myself up to Ori in the kitchen, and he couldn't hear me. And then, he unknowingly gave me the perfect entree to Roth's book when he shouted from the bathroom: "There you go, getting ready to bolt."

And bolt I did; I went to Maine. I found an Airbnb, and I went to a spa. After the spa, I sat at a bar and had a fattening dinner with dessert and a glass of wine. When I went to bed, I tossed and turned all night, looking at my phone, wondering why Ori did not text me his usual "Goodnight." All the while, having listened to three of the five CDs in Roth's book and thinking: "Holy shit, I am an obsessive-compulsive eater, and I spend my days giving myself permission to eat or not eat."

Getting out of food jail

In one of the CDs, she explained that when you can find peace within yourself and stay in the present moment, you no longer have to be "on a diet" and "the weight will naturally fall off." I hate that expression because when I permit myself to eat, my first reaction is to eat candy and carbs, not healthy foods. Permitting myself to eat is like I have been in food jail my whole life, and I am finally free. For me, this release from food jail and being finally free happens every day, three to six times a day. Hence, the obsessive-compulsive hell in which I live.

Shut up, shut up!

In CD #4, Roth talks about not listening to that crazy voice inside your head that is always criticizing you. You know, the one that grabs my stomach every night to see how I have done or the one that undermines my desire to succeed by deciding if I am too fat to be good enough. The voice that can only think about how fat I am when I am trying to meditate. The voice that values my accomplishments by how thin or fat I am. The voice that knows I don't deserve success because I'm fat and, therefore, every investment in my business is potentially a waste of money. Yeah, her.

In CD #4, Roth also says that all compulsive eaters are either restrictors (constantly on a diet) or permittors (always giving permission to binge). A restrictor becomes a permittor when they are bingeing, and a permittor becomes a restrictor when they are dieting. I think I am both, but Roth says you can only be one or the other. Stop the madness! What will I learn on CD #5, the last CD?

What am I surrendering?

I woke up at 2:22 a.m. at the Airbnb and realized that I had not brushed my teeth. The voice inside me said, "You could at least have some discipline in your life and brush your teeth." So I got up and brushed my teeth, and then I started to write this chapter, the one that talks about how surrender is required.

Am I ready to surrender? Maybe, but surrender what? Am I surrendering this voice in my head that has been undermining my entire life? Am I surrendering any temporary pleasure I may get from eating unhealthy food and then the sadistic pleasure I get in beating myself up if I have eaten to a place where I feel sick and then, throwing up?

Am I surrendering the loser who cannot meditate because she continually has to feel her belly for some kind of validation, good or bad? Am I surrendering the woman who blames her husband for her unhappiness? Am I surrendering the woman who is married to a man who may be slightly more miserable than she but thankfully more productive in the world, so there is plenty to eat?

Oh God—or should I say Goddess Sophia—precisely what am I surrendering? I feel as if there is a wall around me that separates me from my success. Therefore, once I remove this shield or the weight, I will be successful—hallelujah!—right? And yet, every day, you, Sophia, share with me grace and magical events in nature to let me know that you are waiting for me. I know you are waiting for me, and I know that I, too, am magical; I know I am the Divine. I just wish this voice in my head would shut up.

I surrender

If *she* shut up, I would be able to stay present and choose healthy foods, and find peace with myself, move my body and connect to my inner divinity. I would be inspired to fulfill my Divine ministry because I motivate myself and shine my inner light out to others. I would stop loathing myself. There ... I said it, I hate this aspect of myself, and I have been at war with her my entire life. Yes, Sophia, I surrender this war inside myself, this mean girl in me, this aspect of me (known as Jersey Girl) that is snarky, destructive, and criticizes Ori and me.

Sophia, please help me to re-direct my energy from that of tearing myself apart to that of motivating me to reach greater heights with my Divine ministry and to fulfill the requests that I receive from Ascended Beings to work on their behalf here on the earth plane. Amen!

Surrender from Recovery

As previously shared, I surrendered my addiction after I received a spiritual message from my grandmother telling me that if I did not stop vomiting, I would die. Yet, even with that powerful message from my grandmother, I had to have one more episode (like just one more drink to an alcoholic). The vomiting ended with a dramatic nosebleed and pain all over my body. It was as if my body had finally said, "ENOUGH!" Thank goodness I listened, and I was ready to be in 100 percent surrender.

What was the difference between the screaming pissed off woman/child described above in *Surrender from Addiction* and the woman who is surrendering and in recovery? The most obvious difference is that I had finally hit rock bottom, and I had nowhere lower to go. I had to choose life over death. I discovered that it was in choosing life that I indeed was in Surrender.

Learning to trust me

I chose to restore my body, to heal the obsessive voices in my head, and to calm my emotions and, most of all, to truly trust that the Divine would have my back. I knew that I could not do this alone, but I also knew that I was the only one who could help me. I had to trust myself first so that I could accept the love and guidance of all of my healing team, my family and friends, and, of course, Sophia. Over the 40-plus years of my struggle, grace was always around me, but I was not ready to receive it. I felt angry, humiliated, embarrassed, shameful, and guilty.

Until I could surrender the madness of my addiction, I could not get well. In fact, I was spiraling towards death. The wounded person described at the beginning of this chapter could not surrender, even though she wrote the words that *sounded* like surrender. The wounded person who could genuinely surrender was the one who chose life over addiction. Sophia was very clear when she shared that she will know when we are genuinely in surrender.

Crossing the bridge

Surrender is the bridge between suffering and grace, and, to be clear, we may not receive the grace we need to stop suffering without first crossing the bridge of surrender. The first part of recovery is where you are climbing out of your ravine of suffering. And then, when you are clearly in surrender, you start making your way down the path to extraordinary grace. In surrender, Sophia sees when you have crossed the middle of the bridge, and you are moving towards grace. This same bridge is the one between human existence and a Divine existence. When you are in grace, you are aware of your Divinity. Now, grace emanates from me, and I am safe and secure in my recovery. Are you ready to receive grace in your life?

Pain is inevitable, suffering is an option, surrender is required, and grace must be allowed. In the next chapter, we will review why someone would or would not allow grace into their lives.

"Sophia, can you give me an example of what the four parts of Sophia's Divine Path to Healing can look like in someone's life?"

She replied, "Imagine sitting on the floor of a dark room, alone and in pain. This scene portrays what suffering feels like. The moment you find the courage to get up and look for the light switch, you are in surrender. When you turn on the light, you are filled with the light of grace. From here, you will find the door that leads you out of the dark room and back into self-love and ultimately, into your Divinely inspired life."

GRACE MUST BE ALLOWED

Defining grace

When Sophia first shared this last step with me, I was intrigued by the language. First, what does "grace" mean, and second, why must grace be allowed? The Hebrew word for grace is *chen*. It is composed of the Hebrew letters *chet* (pictured by a fence, meaning private, or to separate from outside) and *nun* (portrayed by a seed of life or later a fish, meaning activity, life, continue or heir). The word itself means "beauty or loveliness," and literally in the paleo-Hebrew means "to separate from the outside" or "protect life." This single, simple Hebrew word is translated into English using many words, including grace, favor, charm, acceptance, kindness, pleasant, precious, and elegance.

How can a word that means "to separate from the outside" or "protect life" also mean "beauty" or "loveliness"? Grace is the knowledge of our true Oneness, the magnificence of our connection to the Divine. To know this, we must be protected from our separateness. From the moment we are born, we are learning how to be separate from the Divine. Then, we go on our spiritual journey to learn how to come back into union with our Divinity. When you are in a state of addictive behavior, you are not only separate from yourself but, most likely, from all of Creation. You are not living in appreciation of the vast beauty and love that is present in your life. This addictive behavior is perpetuated by a sense of lack of self-worth and connection to self and others.

Defining "grace must be allowed"

Therefore, after you choose not to suffer, and as surrender is required, then grace must be allowed. My interpretation of "grace must be allowed" means you are ready to give up the pain of your addiction. After all, addiction enables you to wallow in your self-pity and be less than productive in your life. It allows you to have an excuse not to speak your truth or stand in your power…an excuse to sell yourself short. As an addict, I did sell myself short. If I sell myself "long," then I must be willing to love myself and others unconditionally. Yeshua defined unconditional love as "acceptance without judgment." Another interpretation of *grace must be allowed* is the idea that I must love myself enough to allow grace to flow to me. Grace is always available, but you need to love yourself enough to let it in.

The way to develop your most robust sense of unconditional love is to separate yourself from the outside world by going inside via prayer or meditation to where you have an unlimited connection to source or grace. Imagine this place, deep inside of you that has the answers and resources that you need for the rest of your life. If that is true, however, then why isn't everyone meditating 24/7? Beyond the practical answer to that question, it is possible that humanity doesn't feel worthy of receiving grace.

Feeling worthy of grace

Oh, boy, there is that word "worthy" again. Self-worth, worthy, deserving of Sophia's grace. Let's be very clear right now, as Divine beings, we are worthy of all that is good and loving. Will there be difficulties and fearful experiences? Of course, because we are still human. Perhaps these experiences are just opportunities to get back in touch with our inner divinity and search for the answers from that place within ourselves. We never know how grace will arrive, and this next story is an example of how grace can arrive.

One day in a healing session, I was taken into a very deep space of healing within myself. I connected with King Solomon and the Queen of Sheba, and I acknowledged their Divine presence. As I went deeper into the meditation, I felt their presence on either side of my head. Then they reached out and adjusted my crown. They did not adjust my crown *chakra* but the etheric golden crown that was sitting on top of my head. I could feel the golden crown on top of my head for the first time!

Then they showed me my beautiful robe of red with white dots and a white fur-like collar. Last, they showed me my lovely golden staff, which was in my left hand. I was surprised to feel these garments and objects, and I was confused as to why I had them. King Solomon spoke and said, "You must step into your queendom, Robin. It is time." In our connection to our true Divine nature, we each become the Queen or King of our own lives.

All hail their own Queen or King

According to Merriam-Webster, the definition of queendom is 1. the state or territory ruled by a queen and 2. the position of a queen. The state or territory that I know I have sovereignty over is my inner world. Therefore, I can be fully connected and in a relationship with my inner queendom. However, to fully be in the position of queen, I must learn to be empowered in my external world as well. The inner world seems more natural to me than the outer world.

Okay, if I am truthful, they are both scary, and I find it hard to commit to both. We only need ten minutes a day, or even fewer, to hear the guidance or truth for our lives. Finding ten minutes is hard, and, like anything else, it requires commitment. It requires the initial uncomfortable element of listening to your mind and then feeling your body. What I know for sure is that the answers to every question for my life are on the inside. Until you are ready to know the answers for your life and forgive yourself and others, it is hard to concentrate while in meditation.

Oprah and Deepak blow my mind

While I was writing this chapter, Oprah and Deepak Chopra gifted their followers with a 21-day meditation called *Manifesting Grace through Gratitude*. I was excited to learn how Oprah and Deepak were going to share more about how Sophia brings us grace. And then Day 2 happened. Here is the write-up:

Day 2: Gratitude Is Within You. Gratitude is a two-way flow of appreciation between your thanks and the uplifting response that you feel in return. Today in our meditation, we begin that conversation and find that as this conversation expands, we create even more thankfulness. We discover how the flow of gratitude from the heart is received by Nature in the same spirit it is given, and it is returned back to us as grace. In today's meditation, we learn to express gratitude from the silence of our awareness, which is the source of grace within.

Wait! Has grace been within me all along? How did I miss that? I missed that because I had been caught in the cycle of victim and victimizer within my addiction. In the chaotic energy of addiction, it is most difficult to feel grace. Yet, even the way I just wrote, "feel grace"—that should have been a big hint that grace was within me all along. For as much as we can abuse ourselves, we can also love ourselves with equal or greater commitment. Once we are in a state of self-love, then we are in gratitude, and then we can feel the grace that has been within us all along.

You are a Divine Spark of God

It is so easy to think of spirituality as a process that is outside of yourself. Just think of the famous quote: "There, but for the grace of God, go I." This quote is a recognition that the misfortune of others could be ours if not for the blessing of the Divine or one's luck. Another interpretation of this quote could be that our fate is in God's hands.

If our fate is in God's hands, then why would we need to learn to love ourselves? Why bother if our destiny is in God's hands. Why not just stay in the throes of addiction? The answer is that the definition above must be expanded to remind us that we are each a Divine Spark of God. If a small spark of God lives within each one of us, then who is responsible for our fate? Is it the God who lives outside of us or the God who lives within us?

Taking grace literally

I further confused the matter for myself by saying that Sophia would *bring us* grace. I believed that right up until I did the Oprah/Deepak meditation program. I considered re-writing the book as a result of my thinking, but I considered that if this was my thought process, then perhaps it may be yours, too. As a society, we often place religious deities, clergy people, and spiritual gurus in between God and us. We don't make it easy to get to God (or to Sophia or Yeshua or any other Ascended Masters.) Yet the path to all of these Beings of Light has always been inside of each of us. The true teaching of grace lies within every one of us.

Does the Divine bring me grace, which I then must recognize and feel inside of myself, or does the Divine spark within me manifest the grace already within me from a place of gratitude? I think the answer is both. As a Divinely guided person, I live in alignment with all of Divinity and with my Divine spark. As a Divine Being, I am responsible for my fate. Which fate will you choose today? You can choose one of self-love and wellness or one of addiction and despair.

Blessing of Love

I invite you to read the following story before making your choice: When I visit my mother and step-father in Florida, I get up every morning to watch the sunrise on the beach, rain or shine. On this particular morning, it was "just" your standard magnificent Florida sunrise that turned into a sunny, clear sky and 70-degree early morning. Feeling underwhelmed, I decided to leave the beach. As I walked up to the path, I said to Yeshua, "This was not a particularly magical morning." Hearing myself, I started to laugh because just being there at that moment of Divine splendor was magnificent, and then I went into sincere gratitude.

I knew Yeshua heard me because I could hear his laughter, too. As I started to walk up the path, a young man of color with long dreadlocks and wearing a hoody came towards me on the one-person path. My reaction was probably typical of many women walking alone: I became scared of what he might do to me.

I asked, "Yeshua, can you walk with me?" At that moment, all of the fear left my being, and it was replaced with the energy of unconditional love (a knowing of acceptance without judgment). I continued on the path and smiled at the young man.

He smiled the most beautiful smile at me and said, "Are you here for the Blessings of Love meeting?"

I replied, "The recovery meeting on the beach or *meeting you*, right here on the path."

He smiled and said, "The one right here on the path. Blessings of Love to you, ma'am."

I replied to him, "Blessings of Love to you, young man."

We both smiled and took a few steps in the directions we were traveling on the path. Then, we both turned and looked back at each other and laughed as we waved "goodbye." Maybe we both turned around at the same time because the encounter felt so magical that we both wanted to make sure that the other was not an angel!

I have often thought about the encounter with this young man on the path. Here he was, heading to an addiction recovery meeting on the beach, and here I was, heading home to be of service to my mother and step-father. He and I were just two recovering addicts filled with the

Blessings of Love on the path between the Divine's magnificent wonders and the responsibilities of everyday life. On the outside, our differences were apparent, but on the inside, our knowing was the same. Recovery from addiction is a journey of excavating the fear from our lives and replacing it with the Blessings of Love available from the Divine. Grace must be allowed. May all your days be filled with Blessings of Love from this day forward.

After I wrote the last four chapters on Sophia's Divine Path to Healing, Yeshua came into my consciousness to tell me that something was missing from the book. What could it be? I invite you to read the next chapter to find out.

"Sophia, why does someone in recovery from addiction feel compelled to continue to describe themselves as an addict?"

"This question has a multi-level response," shared Sophia.

"On the most human level, individuals in recovery are terrified of slipping back into using their addictive substance. Therefore, if they call themselves a recovering addict, they can remind themselves of how far they have come and where they do not want to return. Recovery must take place in many parts of your life, including:

- *staying connected to your Divine nature*

- *healing your past*

- *living in a supportive environment*

- *having a positive mindset*

- *maintaining health and wellness*

- *having solid plans for your present moment and future lifestyle*

Recovery (and ultimately, remission) takes a commitment to not suffering, requires true surrender, and an openness to receiving grace. When you can do these well and live a congruent lifestyle, you are no longer an addict, and you have moved from recovery to remission."

FINDING WHOLENESS

Finding the missing piece

"Something is missing from the book," Yeshua said to me.

I decided to "unbusy" myself to hear what was missing. What could it be? In the spiritual writing process, I have learned to let go and see where the Divine is going to take me. All Yeshua would share with me was one word: "Wholeness."

What is wholeness in the recovery process? On the surface level, it would appear to be a holistic approach to recovery that incorporates mind, body, spirit, and emotion. Eat healthily, take supplements, exercise, go to therapy, meditate, be in nature, change your mindset, receive energy healing, and be in a community of like- minded people.

Could this be *just the beginning* of what is required for long-term recovery? I had posed this question earlier in the book, "Can someone go from recovery to remission?" Perhaps an expanded definition of wholeness is required to make this incredible transition from recovery to remission. Let's follow the breadcrumbs that Yeshua placed out for me.

Carl Jung explains addiction

In the article, *Craving Wholeness: The Complexity of Addiction* by Nina Marie Corona, I discovered information that was very much in alignment with this book. Corona shares,

> Believe it or not, it was a psychologist who deemed addiction a spiritual problem! In the 1930s, Carl Jung worked extensively with a patient who suffered from alcoholism, and after about a year of psychoanalysis, the man relapsed. It was then that Jung determined that psychiatry had been ineffective, and that he believed the man's only hope was a "spiritual awakening" or a "religious experience." Jung later wrote about the man's condition in a letter to Bill Wilson, the co-founder of Alcoholics Anonymous. Jung wrote that his former patient's "craving for alcohol was the equivalent … of the spiritual thirst of our being for wholeness … the union with God." Jung's now-infamous solution was *spiritus contra spiritum*, which loosely translated means: "substitute the spirit of God for the alcoholic spirits." St. Augustine understood this craving long before Jung, and he wrote in his *Confessions* that "this craving or restlessness can be stilled only by God."

Jung's theory was implying that the spirit of alcohol was a misguided attempt to fill an "unrecognized spiritual need," a craving for wholeness, and a desire for connection with others. People use substances to fill a need, and usually, the need can be spiritual. People drink "to feel more connected, more creative, more at peace, less afraid, or more loved." Being high from substances can mimic spiritual states of consciousness and temporarily fill a spiritual void.

Spirit vs. Soul

Reading the article brought me to a dilemma that I was not sure I had the answer to: "What is the difference between Soul and Spirit?" Based on what I read in Corona's writings, it seemed that there was an energy of God that was missing or dormant in an addictive person. As someone who works closely with the Soul energy, I was confident to say that our individual Soul is a Divine Spark of God, our identity, and our unique connection to the overall spirit of all Divinity.

While Soul and Spirit are used interchangeably, Spirit is more of grace-filled energy that fills us and flows in and out of us. Spirit is in constant motion helping us to heal whatever we are committed to healing and bringing us whatever we most desire in life. Why would anyone choose to use false spirits (substances, limiting beliefs, other people's control mechanisms) over the grace-filled Spirit that is available to each of us?

Because of my new state of recovery from food addiction, I realized I was not the expert who could share an expanded version of wholeness. Who could help me to understand this? Of course, it would be one of my favorite spiritual teachers, Carolyn Myss. Yeshua led me to her audiobook *Anatomy of the Spirit*. I listened to this brilliant work on my way to visit friends, and once again, on my way back home.

Divinely inspired listening

When you receive an impulse from the Divine realm to read a book, you do not just read it; you consume it. Every sentence is filled with just what you need to hear. I highly recommend this book for anyone interested in the spiritual path. In it, Carolyn shared that individuals stay in addiction because they are not ready to face the truth of their lives. This truth often is terrifying and takes an incredible commitment to the healing journey. You must be willing to examine your emotions from the past and the present.

I do know what it means to heal on an emotional level. I have spent many healing sessions with professionals and alone with the Divine with deep grief coming up through my chakra system and having that grief getting caught in the fifth chakra, my will center. In the process, I would be choking on my grief until I took control of my panic and started breathing through my nose, allowing the grief to leave my throat in a tortured cry. This process allowed me to extinguish the emotional charges from my original trauma, free up the stuck energy in my body, open up my throat chakra to then be able to cry out my truth and then activate my will to heal fully. This type of healing is not for the faint of heart—but maybe, just maybe, it is for you.

Anatomy of the Spirit

For those of you who may be unfamiliar with the chakra system, the chakras are energy storage centers within our physical vessel. They are our power centers. These power centers must remain open, spinning, and clear of any psychic debris in order for you to manage your power. In *Anatomy of the Spirit*, Myss compares the chakra system to the Christian sacraments and the Judaic Kabbalah Tree of Life. In essence, she is showing how the Divine teachings are alive and well within our physical vessel.

In *Anatomy of the Spirit*, Myss also explains that our fourth chakra (the heart chakra) must come into <u>congruence</u> with our sixth chakra (the mind chakra) to activate our fifth chakra (the throat chakra), our *will* center. In an interview in *Unity Magazine* by Katy Koontz, Myss describes "congruence" as follows:

> Congruent means that what you say, what you think, and what you do are in alignment with your spiritual and soul values, so they all work together. To me, *authentic* is like a noun—you can say something is authentic, and it stops there. Congruent is like a verb because it's an ongoing practice of moving into alignment. To be congruent, you have to put effort into paying attention to the relationship between what you think, say, and do.

Myss shares the following guidelines to practice spiritual congruence:

- You should say only what you believe and believe what you say.
- Power originates behind your eyes, not in front of your eyes. True power is invisible.

- Thought precedes the creation of matter. Every thought is a tool. Every thought is a prayer.
- Judgment anchors you to the person or thing you judge, making you its servant.

The key to success

Being congruent is the key to long-term success in recovery; it's the answer to how to move to remission ultimately. When you are congruent (when your heart, your mind, <u>and</u> your body are on the same page, and you are no longer undermining yourself), you can activate your will center, which we also refer to as your "will power." When you have reliable will power, then even the hardest situations cannot throw you out of recovery.

When you are congruent, you will have worked hard to ground your Soul energy in your physical vessel. When you are congruent, you can recognize the Spirit that flows in and out of you; the grace that is your birthright. Grace flows in for you to heal; grace flows out for you to help others heal.

Developing your spiritual will

The last article I was drawn to read was an article housed on *visionarylead. org*. The article gave me a deep understanding of the different levels of the power of will. In *Developing Your Spiritual Will* by Corinne McLaughlin and Gordon Davidson, they define what will is and the different levels of will. The authors shared:

> The will is the directive and regulatory function in your life; it balances and constructively utilizes all your energies. On a deeper level, will is related to the life principle – it brings life to an individual or an organization. On a deeper metaphysical level, it is synonymous with the breath. Will is also a clarifying, purifying energy, needed to destroy old forms before new forms can be built. The aspects of will are dynamic energy, persistence, determination,

and one-pointedness. To be effective, the will also has to be skillful, not just powerful. When rightly used, will is expressed with love and understanding and is dedicated to the purposes of Light. It is used to destroy all that hinders the free flow of human life. The use of pure will is only possible for a coordinated thinker.

The article included the stages of developing your will that you can encounter on your path to wholeness:

Personal Will: The first step in developing a spiritual will is developing discipline and focus. By creating goals and standards for what is essential for your life and holding your standards with impeccable integrity, you will manifest what you most desire in your life.

Goodwill: The next step is developing a charitable purpose and a benevolent disposition towards others. Goodwill expresses compassion, generosity, and forgiveness, and it nourishes the spirit of understanding and cooperation. Goodwill is our first attempt to express the love of God.

Embodying God's Will: This is the final step when you renounce your personal will and become a stream of Universal will or Divine will. By submitting to Divine will and merging with it, you gain clear intention and Divine purpose. Persistence is your power state.

Gaining congruence

As I waited patiently to "receive" the right content for this missing chapter, Yeshua shared with me, "*Feast & Famine* is the first book of a trilogy with *Messiah Within* being the second and *The Divine Keys* being the third."

I replied, "That's interesting since I am writing *Feast & Famine* last."

He replied, "That is because you were not ready to write *Feast & Famine*, but you were ready to work with the Divine when I came to you to write the other two books."

I interpreted this to mean that I first had *Divine Will,* then I had *Goodwill,* and lastly, I developed *Personal Will.*

Why did I live this trilogy of will backward? The answer is simple: I wrote and published the first two books as an addict and with a dysfunctional personal will. Therefore, I could never stand behind the first two books with congruence, which requires *personal will.* In recovery from addiction, with my heart, mind, and body in full alignment and with a healthy trilogy of will, I could now live my Soul Mission and present the book trilogy to the world.

When you choose to live in congruence, you will be able to heal your addiction with grace and recognize the real purpose of your life. When you allow grace into your life, you will discover that even in your darkest moments, you were never alone. And now, in your moments of most magnificent light, you will recognize that you are an integral part of all life. Welcome home. Welcome to wholeness.

As a congruent being, you can safely move into a phase of self-transformation that will be powerful and effective. In the next chapter, you will discover how to forgive all aspects of yourself.

"Sophia, I was inspired to look up the word "junkie" and found this description in the Urban Dictionary. A junkie is a person who is consumed by an addiction. Aspects of their life suffer as he/she satisfies the addiction.

Let me see if I can re-word the definition Sophia-style: A junkie is a person who is consumed with suffering. Aspects of their life are consumed by addiction as he/she satisfies their choice to suffer."

Sophia exclaimed, "Exactly! That is a more accurate description from our viewpoint!"

THE RETIRED JUNKIE

From fear to purpose

When I was struggling mightily with my bulimia, I asked my spiritual best friend, "Why am I still struggling with bulimia?"

She replied, "Because you are a junkie."

Being a junkie would imply that I was still in the throes of my addiction and either struggling to quit or not able to quit. After about a thousand different attempts to stop, it was clear that I just didn't know how to stop the pattern. I certainly knew the "right" actions to take, but I was scared. What could I be so afraid of? After lifetimes of persecution, I was scared of everything. Who could blame me?

By following Sophia's Divine Path to Healing, I am finally living my mission as a Divine Emissary, a person who integrates the spiritual teachings and then lives them without concern for what others will think or whether it is safe to share his or her message. I have a message to share; in fact, I have many messages to share. How can I let a "little" problem liked being killed by an angry mob in a past life stop me from speaking the Divine truth?

The protective addict

I had invited the Addict archetype to bring me to such lows that I would have no choice but to heal both my past and current lifetimes. Instead of being angry at my junkie, I started to appreciate the role it has played as my grand protector. My junkie protected me from experiencing current and past life traumas over and over again in this lifetime. My junkie acted in what has been the traditional masculine role in our society: to serve and protect and to provide resources.

Is the Addict archetype also a shield for incredibly brilliant and powerful Soul energy? Are junkies afraid to shine their Light out into the world? If we don't shine our Light, then we are still hiding in the shadows. I came out of the spiritual closet many years ago, but now I realize it was not in all my brilliance.

Welcoming the masculine

I know I must live at my highest vibration and in integrity with my messenger mission for this lifetime. My junkie masculine will retire from its protective service when I am placing my purpose at the front of my priorities. To be clear, I am not asking the masculine to retire from my life; in fact, I am calling my Divine Masculine to return to manifest an extraordinary life in concert with my magnificent Divine Feminine.

I also forgive my junkie masculine for all the lifetimes that it fell short on its mission, and I died an untimely death because of it. I forgive the people in my lifetimes to whom I looked for filling this role for me, and they failed. I forgive myself for bringing in a junkie masculine energy to protect myself in this lifetime from my deep fear of persecution.

One day at a time

By shining my light as bright and far as I can, I am Grace, and Grace is me. Will I have difficult days? You bet! When my junkie returns intermittently, as it inevitably will at times, it will be a reminder that

I have work to do that is incredibly essential. In mindful reflection at those times, perhaps I will realize that I am just bored and looking for food to fill me up. I will say thank you to my junkie for the reminder to get busy, or I will gently reply to my junkie that I am choosing to relax, and I will get busy soon enough. Either way, ironically, my junkie has become my hero, my protector, and I love it with all my heart.

I invite you, dear reader, to bring forth both your Divine Feminine and Divine Masculine energies into your day-to-day life. Take the time to discover where these powerful energies are in alignment with your highest good and where they may be undermining your success. When you can recognize both the light and the shadow in your life and take steps to heal your life, your life will become a series of magical moments. In the perfect alignment of your Divine Feminine and Divine Masculine, you will become creative, compassionate, loving, and kind, actively serving yourself and others, and manifesting the life of your dreams. That is your Divine Right.

"If you want to awaken all of humanity, then awaken all of yourself. If you want to eliminate the suffering of the world, then eliminate all that is dark and negative in yourself. Truly, the greatest gift you have to give is that of your own self-transformation." Lao Tzu

This book would not be complete without the wisdom of people who are deeply spiritual and in long-term recovery. After all, they are truly walking the walk. Turn to the next chapter to read more.

Sophia's Insights for Chapter Eighteen

"Sophia, why did you think it was important to include in this book the opinions of individuals who have been on their recovery and remission journeys from suffering?" I asked.

Sophia replied, "The intention is to give past, present, and future view of addiction from individuals whom you chose who were both in long-term recovery and were deeply spiritual. What did you find the most interesting about the survey results?"

I replied, "I discovered that none of them would change anything about their past, which was filled with addiction, because they would not have become the person they are now. Learning this just gave me such great hope for myself and all addicts."

"Indeed, there is great hope and love for all," shared Sophia.

CHAPTER EIGHTEEN

THE LONG VIEW

Throughout my journey of addiction and spirituality, I have often met people who survived powerful addictions, maintained long-term recovery, and became deeply spiritual. Beyond being in awe of them, I was curious to know their long-term perspective so that I could share it with you. Since I was in my first year of recovery while re-writing this book, I did not have direct experience of long-term success. I hope that their words will inspire you to stay the course of your recovery. I asked each of the responders the same ten questions.

1. **What substance or set of actions did you use that would feed your addiction?**

   The most predominant answer was alcohol, which makes a lot of sense since it is so readily available and glamorized in our entertainment industry. As someone who has a few glasses of wine every year, I find it so interesting that many TV shows feature alcohol as a way to celebrate success or heal from disappointment.

   One of the recipients responded that her first drug of choice was sweet foods that were forbidden at home. Then, when she could drink legally at eighteen, she jumped right on the alcohol wagon.

   Another responder said that she went from alcohol to a host of narcotics as she wanted a different kind of high. Thinking back to what Sophia has shared, there is no high from food, alcohol, or drugs that can remove the suffering since the problem is the suffering itself. Sobriety must occur first before the suffering can be healed.

2. **Do you think you became addicted to a substance or action, or was your addiction to the act of suffering?**

I was curious to hear their answers as this concept was new to me when I wrote the book. And not surprisingly, I did not truly get a response to the question. The most relevant answer was, *"I have finally acknowledged that I was traumatized as a very young child. A child cannot possibly deal with or process trauma, so I turned to food to survive, to push the feelings down because if I felt the feelings, they would overwhelm and kill me. Alcohol was the next logical step."*

The rest of the answers were centered around how alcohol and drugs were both a physical and emotional addiction. I would agree with them but as a second-level addiction. Their suffering was their first-level addiction.

3. **What triggered your desire to stop your addiction? Did it feel that you had hit your rock bottom?**

In reading the responses, what stood out for me was how each person said that the act of drinking or doing drugs took center stage in their lives. Even if they were working or doing something else, they would be thinking about their next high. Many were lonely and afraid, and the alcohol made them more social and likable.

This following answer particularly hit home for me, thinking back on all of the times that I would sneak out of the house to get copious amounts of snacks to eat obsessively. *"When I couldn't stand myself anymore, I would drive to San Antonio to drink with friends there, and then I participated in more abusive behavior that made me hate myself even more. It is a vicious cycle that you think will be fixed with the very substance that causes the hell. It was a huge amount of pain and suffering physically, spiritually, emotionally, and mentally."*

4. **Did you have to surrender to a higher power to enter recovery?
    What was your process?**

The answers to this question had a similar theme: to stop suffering
and to stop using their chosen poison; they had to surrender.
Whether it was to a higher power we know as God or to a higher
power via a therapist or the squirrel in one person's back yard, the
path to recovery began with a powerful act of surrender. From this
surrender, the grace arrived in a different package, depending on
what their needs were. However, what I admired most about their
answers is that to attain a long-term result, they were required to
learn to love themselves.

Here is an example: *"It was an incredibly spiritual process of going
within to find my Source and Higher Power. I had to rethink ALL of
my beliefs and replace them with new and positive affirmations. After
34 years clean and sober, I am STILL in the process of growing and
evolving. I've never stopped being teachable as I expand my Higher
Self in all ways possible. The most important part of my growth was
learning to feel my feelings, so I didn't have to use substances anymore."*

5. **Has your definition of a higher power changed over time, from
    an external view to an internal view?**

When I first became interested in spirituality, I was curious to
understand the difference between spirituality and religion. While
both paths can lead you to the Divine, the main distinction for
me became this: that religion is an outward-facing vehicle, and
spirituality is an inward-facing vehicle. In essence, in religion, God
is outside of you; in spirituality, God is inside you. The answers to
the survey question truly supported this idea.

a. One of the responders shared, *"Religion is for people who believe
    in Hell; Spirituality is for people who have BEEN to Hell. I know
    the way I acted, thought, and believed led me to one hell of an
    awful way of life and that I was slowly killing myself. Over the*

last several years, however, I have come to believe that the life I choose to create is an inside job. This viewpoint has been helped by the fact that I have not ever had a vision of an omnipotent or punishing 'God.' That has never felt 'right' to me. Why would an entity that touts 'Love' bring terrible things upon me? I now believe that I have the power to live the life I want, as long as I am willing to put in the work and be the best sober person I can be."

b. A beautiful memory was shared by one of the responders: *"I had a life-changing experience at ten months sober. I used to pray to a God that I learned about in the Catholic church. I prayed for peace and acceptance of who I was. I prayed for the health and wellness of my friends and family. I prayed for the world and for those who continued to suffer in it. Then one day, as I was reading poetry at night, I felt an overwhelming feeling of acceptance and self-love. I began to cry, but I couldn't identify what I was feeling. I was moved to get on my knees and thank God.*

While I was there crying and feeling all the love, I realized the whole room was FILLED to the walls with the beautiful LOVE. It was pressing all around me and expanded out through the walls. When I began to look for the Source, I realized it was coming from ME! I was shocked and amazed because I had always thought God was outside of me, and now I knew for sure that this Source was a part of me, inside me. I was blessed. I sobbed and gave thanks. I know now. I am God. A beautiful tiny spark of God, and so is everyone else on the planet. We are all part of God, and we are ONE."

6. Have you healed your original trauma(s) related to your trigger(s) for addiction? If so, how?

As you might have guessed, healing your childhood or teen traumas can take a long time and a sincere dedication to your long-term sobriety. What I have discovered in my healing journey is that our wounded child inside will stay with us, protecting us from further harm, until we are ready to move beyond the hurt to a healthy acceptance of what has transpired in our lives. Once our wounded inner child knows that we are doing just fine, she/he will integrate back into our full psyche. This process takes patience and often professional support to achieve. Here are three of the responses received in the survey:

a. *"I let my inner child know that she is safe, that what happened was WRONG, that SHE is not wrong, she is wonderful and amazing and fantastic. As an adult, I still find those words hard to believe, but I continue to do self-esteem and self-love work through books, meditations, and journaling."*

b. *"Being accountable for my actions rather than feeling like the victim or without a sense of control of my own life brings serenity and grounding, which are necessary for mental and emotional stability. All things needed to maintain sobriety. I have maintained sobriety through meetings, maintaining a support network with other alcoholics and therapy."*

c. *"Through the Grace of God and the Fellowship of AA, I haven't found it necessary to take a drink or a drug since February 3, 1985, and for that, I am truly grateful. I believe the healing came through reprogramming my internal belief system, turning my life over to the care of my God, forgiving those who hurt me, including myself, and making amends to those I had harmed. My continued sobriety is contingent on my spiritual and emotional health. I meditate every day, no matter what, and I have a support network that I stay connected to that helps me deal with daily trials and trauma. Plus, I give to others whenever I possibly can by coaching, empathizing, and loving others every day."*

7. **Do you believe that there is a cure for addiction based on the following definition?**

A cure has been previously defined in the book as a substance or procedure that ends a medical condition, such as a medication, a surgical operation, a change in lifestyle, or even a philosophical mindset that helps end a person's sufferings; or the state of being healed or cured. This question provided me with a plethora of diverse answers for sure.

As noted earlier in the book, none of the medical or psychological materials support a cure for addiction. Yet, the Divine realm believes that we can be healed or cured if we get to the root of our suffering, then alleviate our pain and, of course, change our lifestyle.

Here is an interesting response: *"I believe that if I start thinking I am 'CURED,' I will feel compelled to 'test the waters' and might decide I can drink. That's the Catch 22 of alcoholism...I have a disease that works very hard to convince me that I don't have a disease. Being very 'mindful' is so in vogue right now, to 'be in the moment' and 'live in the moment' and to 'be present', but that's how I've lived a sober life for 29 years...all I have is right now, today. Tomorrow is not guaranteed, so I want to make the best of today."*

What I find the most interesting about her response is that she is 29 years sober, and she chooses <u>not</u> to say that she is cured —

even though she meets the criteria as defined. If someone was in remission from cancer for 29 years, would they declare they were healed? The art of suffering is so influential that it can genuinely haunt our everyday lives.

8. **Do you believe it is possible to move from recovery to remission from addiction? If so, what standards must you maintain to be in remission?**

I knew this question would stir up the hornet's nest for sure! Moving from recovery to remission means that you have total control over your suffering and your suffering tools. That takes an incredible amount of self-control and sincere devotion to your Divinity. In essence, to enter remission, you must change your mindset from "Suffering is an Option," to "Suffering is No Longer an Option."

Is it possible to get so far ahead of the "disease" that it cannot catch up with you and take over ever again? Not likely, according to most of my responders who are still dependent upon their external power to be an intermediary between them and their addictive behavior. One brave responder who is a deeply internally focused person said quite simply, *"Yes, remission from addiction is abstinence."*

9. **How important is spirituality in your process? What is required to live a life of grace versus a life of suffering?**

One of my favorite parts of writing this book was discovering that grace was both an inside and an outside job. At first, I thought it had to be brought to me by the Divine, but after listening to the Oprah and Deepak meditation (which I mentioned in Chapter Fifteen), I had an aha moment that all of the grace I may ever need resides inside of me. Two answers to this survey question truly moved me.

a. *"Spirituality is the foundation of my process. Most importantly, to have gratitude. I am sincerely grateful that I wake up, and my eyes open every single day. I can get myself out of bed, and I have an indoor bathroom with everything I could possibly need. I don't take anything for granted. I also deeply APPRECIATE everything in my life, even the not-so-great stuff. The most important thing is that I'm alive and sober. Everything else is just 'stuff.'"*

b. *"It is the most important part of my process. There are no requirements to live a life of grace except to recognize who you truly are and own it/accept it. I am a child of God. I still suffer sometimes because I am also human. But if I stay connected to others who love me, and I continue to love and take care of myself, then I have so much grace, it's not even funny. It's a miracle. There is no more suffering in my life except for my ego, who is emotionally attached to something that gets taken away. The good thing is that I can separate myself from my ego and see it for what it is and know that this, too, shall pass."*

10. If you could have a conversation with your younger self about the addiction cycle, what would you tell them about your experience in addiction, recovery, and remission that could change their mindset and place them on a different path?

After I got the survey results back, I remember being pleasantly shocked that most of the responders would not tell their younger selves anything to change their path. They felt they would not be the person they are today without the experiences they had in the past. I was sure they were going to respond differently. Yet, it gave me such hope for anyone reading this book who is considering or already in surrender. It reminded me that we don't need to beat ourselves up over our past mistakes because all of our experiences serve the greater good of our Soul's journey in this lifetime. Amen to you, responders — you truly made a difference in my life. Here are some of their inspiring responses.

a. *"I don't know that I could have said anything to my younger self to convince me that there was another way. I believe I got sober when I did because I was ready. It was a 'right time, right place' situa-*

tion. As we say in AA, "I chose to get off the elevator where I did, Ladies Lingerie. I could have gone all the way to the basement, but I decided to get off that ride."

b. *"I would tell my younger self that I don't have to believe the things I was made to believe ... that I was less than enough, not good enough, not important enough."*

c. *"I don't think I would change a thing since it got me to where I am today. Sometimes you have to live life to learn from it."*

d. *"I would try and save myself from all the pain, but the pain has brought me to the place I am now. I wonder if I would be closed, self-centered, without the grace of God if I was never an alcoholic."*

e. *"I would tell my younger me that self-esteem comes from doing estimable acts."*

f. *"I would never do that. I love the path that I took because it brought me to where I am. If I had a conversation with my younger self, I would tell her it's all okay. It's going to be okay. Trust in the process of Life to bring you all you need when you need it. It's all going to turn out just fine. But I wouldn't try to get her to take another path. I've learned to love every bit of hell I went through because it helps me to relate to others so I can help them in this life. That is my purpose: to help others get on the other side of hell and into the miracle of knowing that we are sparks of the Divine, and we can create heaven on earth. It's true."*

Thank you to the wonderful and wise individuals who answered the survey questions. I am hopeful that their answers inspire anyone who is suffering and in addiction to seek the steps required to come into long-term recovery.

WORDS OF WISDOM AND HOPE

As I was finishing writing *Feast & Famine*, I was guided to read, *The Choice* by Dr. Edith Eva Eger. This book is about Dr. Eger's family experience in Auschwitz. It's about survival for Dr. Eger and how she dedicated her life to helping others who have suffered significant trauma to make other choices. What enabled her to live through the degradation and trauma of Auschwitz was something her mother had said to her before they arrived at the concentration camp on the train.

"Dicuka," her mother said into the darkness one night, "listen. We don't know where we're going. We don't know what's going to happen. Just remember, no one can take away from you what you put into your mind." Dr. Eger shares in her book that it was her ability to imagine a future outside of the horrors of Auschwitz that enabled her to survive.

I devoured this excellent book not only because of my past life relatability but because of the outstanding suggestions for healing that Dr. Eger presents from sessions with her many clients. To say that Dr. Eger's writings have inspired me to keep going is an understatement. She showed me that when you tell your truth, you can have a dramatic impact on the lives of others as well.

I discovered this book on Oprah's *Super Soul Sunday* show, where Dr. Eger was a guest.

Oprah said, "Hello, Dr. Eger."

She replied, "Hello."

She had me at "Hello." I didn't even need to watch the interview; I immediately bought her book. After I finished reading it, I then went back and watched the interview, perhaps saving the best for last!

What I have learned from all of the heroes in my life (including Dr. Eger and Oprah), is that I do have choices. I have a choice to be in recovery, to be healthy, to be wise, and to share Sophia's Divine Path to Healing with you. Yes, your Soul does guide your life, but you also have free will. I invite you to exercise your free will to choose your recovery and to choose serving others by sharing your grace-filled story. Your story may just be what inspires another person who is suffering to make the right choice.

My Dear Ones:

As you come to the end of this book, I am delighted to know that you have read these powerful words intended to heal you from your journey of suffering. Robin was at first a reluctant messenger because she was caught in the throes of her addictive behavior. Over time and with help, she was able to transform herself into the Divine messenger that you have experienced in this book.

I see the possibilities of your life. Yes, you have made mistakes and made bad choices. From my perspective, it has always been your life unfolding in perfect order. That was then, and this is now. Now, you are here, and you are listening. I invite you to forgive yourself for your perceived past transgressions.

Real transformation for your life can only take place in the present moment. When you live in regret of your past or are fearful of your future, you are wallowing in suffering. You must choose a life of surrender and grace. Are you ready to do so? I am ready to hear your heartfelt surrender and to guide you to the grace you need to heal.

What will grace look like for you? That all depends on what you need. Make a list of what you need and share it with me in your prayers. The grace may arrive in a different package than what you had in mind, so do not be tied to any outcomes. Keep doing your work, and I will do my part.

It all begins and ends with your unwavering commitment to your wellness and your service to others.

May your light shine brightly for all beings whom you meet on your path.

In light and love,

Sophia

About the Author

Robin Clare worked for 25 years in corporate America and non-profit administration. Even then, she had a deep passion for spirituality and wellness. In her corporate life, she yearned to live a life where she could be her true authentic self. Robin's path to becoming a Divine Emissary began by leaving her traditional business career to become her authentic spiritual self.

This commitment to her spiritual journey led her to understand her Soul Mission. Robin traveled across the globe to study with spiritual masters and grow into her Divine gifts. Becoming truly authentic required Robin to share her deepest secret. For most of her adult life, Robin struggled with food addiction and bulimia.

She dug deep into her current and past lives to heal the wounds that were blocking her success and keeping her in active addiction. Now, in recovery, she is living her Soul Mission as an author, teacher, and life and business coach. Robin was named Best10 Life/Business Coach and Best10 Energy Healer in the *Natural Nutmeg* 2017, 2018, and 2019 Readers Poll.

Robin has documented her extraordinary spiritual journey in her highly acclaimed books, *Messiah Within* and the Amazon Best-Selling Spiritual book, *The Divine Keys*. Now, she continues to share her journey in *Feast & Famine*.